Field Training Officer

Tips and Techniques for FTOs, Preceptors, and Mentors

Bruce Nepon, MA Ed, NREMT-P
Acting Department Chair, Allied Health
Delaware Technical and Community College
Dover, Delaware

Barry Eberly, NREMT-P, AA
Department of EMS Education
Bayhealth Medical Center
Dover, Delaware

JONES & BARTLETT
LEARNING

World Headquarters
Jones & Bartlett Learning
5 Wall Street
Burlington, MA 01803
978-443-5000
info@jblearning.com
www.jblearning.com

Jones and Bartlett's books and products are available through most
bookstores and online booksellers. To contact Jones and Bartlett
Learning directly, call 800-832-0034, fax 978-443-8000, or visit our
website www.jblearning.com.

Production Credits
Chief Executive Officer: Clayton Jones
Chief Operating Officer: Don W. Jones, Jr.
President, Higher Education and
  Professional Publishing: Robert W. Holland, Jr.
V.P., Sales and Marketing: William J. Kane
V.P., Design and Production: Anne Spencer
V.P., Manufacturing and Inventory Control: Therese Connell
Publisher-Public Safety Group: Kimberly Brophy
Acquisition Editor-EMS: Christine Emerton

Senior Production Editor: Susan Schultz
Director of Marketing: Alisha Weisman
Composition: Cape Cod Compositors
Cover and Text Design: Anne Spencer
Senior Photo Researcher and
  Photographer: Kimberly Potvin
Cover and Interior Photographs: Courtesy of Bruce Nepon,
  Delaware Technical and Community College
Printing and Binding: Edwards Brothers Malloy
Cover Printing: Edwards Brothers Malloy

Library of Congress Cataloging-in-Publication Data:
Nepon, Bruce.
   Field training officer : tips and techniques for FTOs, preceptors, and mentors / Bruce Nepon, Barry Eberly.
   p. cm.
   ISBN 0-7637-4199-X (pbk.)
   1. Emergency medical services—Study and teaching. 2. Emergency medical personnel—Training of. I. Eberly, Barry. II. Title.
   [DNLM: 1. Emergency Medical Services. 2. Emergency Medical Technicians—education. 3. Preceptorship-methods.
   4. Teaching—methods. WX 18 N441f 2007]
   RA645.5.N37 2007
   362.18076-dc22
                                                                                                    2007016813
6048
Printed in the United States of America
19 18 17 16 15   10 9 8 7 6

Contents

Acknowledgments

We gratefully acknowledge the support of the people and organizations listed below. Their assistance was vital to the development of our Field Training Officer workshop presentations.

We first thank our employer. Administrative officers of Bayhealth Medical Center provided invaluable advice and support. We offer a singular thank you to Mr. Al Pilong.

We thank the Delaware Office of Emergency Medical Services (OEMS). The OEMS supported the concept of teaching students to be "team leaders." The OEMS saw value in the development of a Field Training Officer (FTO) workshop. They supported the concept that a properly prepared FTO is more effective than an untrained FTO. Steve Blessing has provided a sense of perspective and direction. The support of the OEMS is greatly appreciated.

We thank Delaware Technical and Community College (DTCC) for giving us an opportunity to refine our model of instruction and evaluation. Feedback from DTCC staff and students has made it possible for us to continue fine-tuning our approach.

We thank the paramedic field training officers of New Castle County EMS, Kent County Paramedics, and Sussex County Paramedics for their thoughtful application of our approach and for their feedback.

We thank the EMS training officers of the Philadelphia Fire Department, Aetna Hose, Hook, and Ladder Company, Harrington Fire Company, and Five Points Fire Company. Feedback received from these agencies allowed us to continue improving our Field Training Officer workshop program.

The following EMS educators provided information about their EMS systems, snapshot views of their various philosophies for EMS instruction, and survey

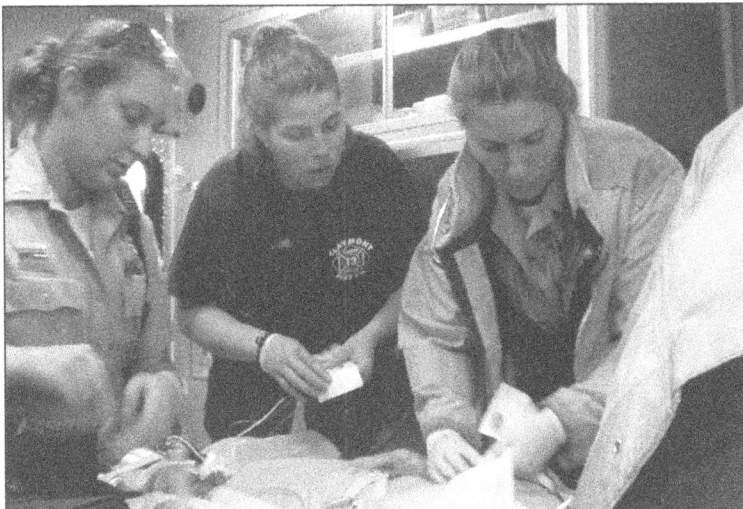

Courtesy of New Castle Emergency Medical Services

responses to several key questions. Their responses provided the authors a better sense of which topics might offer the most potential benefit for FTOs, preceptors, and mentors. We thank the following individuals for their assistance:

Gordon A. Kokx, BS, NREMT-P, Associate Professor, EMS Program Director, The College of Southern Idaho, Twin Falls, Idaho

Rosemary McGinnis, RN, BSN, TNS, EMS System Coordinator and Lead Instructor, Community Hospital Of Ottawa, Ottawa, Illinois

William M. Mehbod, BS, EMT-P, Classroom Coordinator, Bethesda Paramedic Training Program, Bethesda North Hospital, Cincinnati, Ohio

Sean Obrien, AS, NREMT-P, EMS-I, Captain of Educational and Outreach Services, New Britain Emergency Medical Services, New Britain, Connecticut

Kenneth J. Sternig, MS, BSN, EMTP, Milwaukee County EMS Center, Milwaukee, Wisconsin

Michael Touchstone, BS, EMT-P, Fire Paramedic Services Chief, Philadelphia Fire Department, Philadelphia, Pennsylvania

Last, but certainly not least, we thank our families for their patience and support.

Reviewers

Art Breault, NREMT-P, RN, CEN, Albany Medical Center, Albany, New York

Linda Swisher, Sarasota, Florida

Thomas Dibernardo, Sunrise Fire Department and Broward Community College, Ft. Lauderdale, Florida

Beth Ann McNeill, Monroe Community College, Rochester, New York

Sarah Walsh, Mecklenburg EMS Agency, Charlotte, North Carolina

Samuel S. Barnes, MEDIC, Charlotte, North Carolina

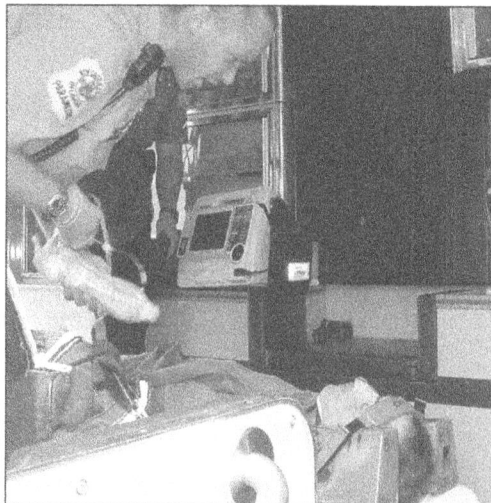

Courtesy of New Castle Emergency Medical Services

Preface

When we began as preceptors in EMS education, neither of us received any guidance as to *how* to perform the job effectively. Although we each had 10 years of experience as field training officers, when we finally did receive some direction, it was simply too subjective to be fair to the students, or to us. The guidance was vague, it did not include concrete guidelines for us to follow in order to be effective teachers and evaluators, and it frequently delayed interventions on the premise that we were operating on a "training unit."

Ten years ago, we began our efforts to resolve these issues. We believe that our Field Training Officer (FTO) workshops, and this text based on those workshops, are a tangible solution to the problems we both saw with regard to preparation of field trainers. We have used the approach described in the text since 1998. It has helped train EMTs and paramedics in college, hospital, fire department, and third-service programs.

This text is intended for field training officers, preceptors, coaches, mentors, instructors, or any EMS personnel who provide instruction and evaluation of patient care providers in the field, clinic, or lab settings. Although we have provided content in the appendices to assist with conducting a field internship, this is not intended for EMS program coordinators or managers as a guide for proper oversight of an EMS program's clinical or field training portions. However, coordinators and managers will find the text useful. It provides forms and documents that can be a reasonable starting point in developing a field internship program.

Throughout the course of this book, the female form (she, her) has been assigned to the FTO. The male form (he, his) has been assigned to the student. This was done simply to provide a format that would be consistent from beginning to end. No other meaning is intended.

This text is not intended to be an encyclopedia of approaches to field training. It is also not intended to present the content as the only method one must use to provide field training. Quite the contrary, the purpose of this text is to share with our colleagues in EMS the lessons we have learned about field training. Our intent is to offer tips and techniques that we have found to be successful when training and evaluating students and providers alike, and to help you avoid the land mines that we have stepped on along the way. Enjoy.

Introduction

This book contains a variety of tips and techniques that experienced field training officers (FTOs) can use to supplement teaching methods they are currently using. New FTOs can use these same tips and techniques to develop an effective approach to teaching and evaluating students that will help them "hit the ground running" as they assume their new duties.

An FTO's duties differ from those of an EMS provider. This text is designed to help FTOs effectively fulfill the roles and responsibilities associated with clinical instruction.

Historically, the change in job classification from provider to FTO was often a sudden event. One day you are an EMT-B or EMT-P, and the next day a student arrives bearing a packet of forms and . . . Surprise! *You* are now the FTO. You would receive the simplest of instructions: "Let us know when you think this student is ready to begin working on his own!"

Thankfully, this situation is becoming less commonplace. Many EMS systems now have written performance standards that define the objectives a student must fulfill before becoming a certified provider. These standards give FTOs a good idea of what their students will be required to accomplish. Unfortunately, these standards frequently do not include a description of instructional techniques the FTO can use to become a more effective teacher.

This lack of guidance often leaves a number of questions unanswered. Questions like: "How much instruction should I provide?" "Will my methods of instruction be effective?" "How can I best evaluate student performance?" "Will I be fair?" "Will my approach be consistent with the methods of my fellow FTOs?" *Field Training Officer* can serve as a resource for the FTO to use to answer these questions.

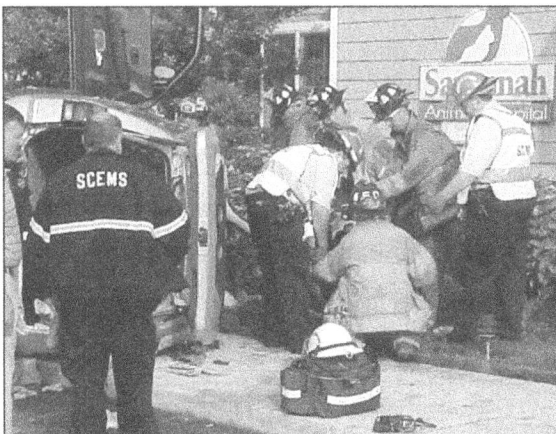

Courtesy of Sussex County EMS

Key Terms

Certain words, terms, and abbreviations occur frequently within the text:

candidate Employee receiving instruction and evaluation during a field internship program.

competency group Subsection of a critique form used to document performance of similar, or related, skills.

critique (form) Form used to document field instruction and field evaluation.

documentation Written evaluation of student performance. Written record of instruction provided to a student.

Field Training Officer (FTO) Used interchangeably with instructor, preceptor, and mentor.

manual A document that describes the field internship process, including written performance standards for students and FTOs (i.e., *Manual for Paramedic Students and FTOs*).

patient contact All assessment and treatment interactions occurring during the care of one patient. Begins at time of dispatch and ends with transfer of patient care.

provider Emergency Medical Technician (EMT-B, EMT-I, or EMT-P).

satisfactory Acceptable student performance.

skill Task a student performs during a patient contact.

student Person receiving instruction and evaluation as part of EMS education.

team leader Student or employee responsible for all aspects of patient care.

unsatisfactory Unacceptable student performance.

Building Blocks for the Field Training Officer: Laying the Groundwork

1

KEY POINTS

- The field training officer is an authority figure.
- Authority is counterbalanced by responsibility.
- High-quality instruction results from the use of effective teaching strategies.

The transition from provider to field training officer (FTO) results in an increase in both authority and responsibility, and these changes are likely to leave most FTOs wondering where to start. The objective of this chapter is to present FTOs with a few tools they can use to build a foundation from which to effectively teach and evaluate students. FTOs will be able to lay this groundwork more easily by anticipating a few of the situations or obstacles that may be encountered.

The FTO as Authority Figure

The first major change for FTOs is obvious: No longer are they just "one of the gang"; the FTO is now an authority figure. The FTO has become one of the decision makers. Interactions with coworkers are likely to take on a completely different tone from anything the FTO has experienced in the past.

Although the new FTO can make every effort to be the same person she was as a field medic, some interactions will be inherently different. The FTO now has the power to make decisions that can have long-term effects on the EMS agency. The FTO will be making decisions about who stays and works and who is not capable of providing EMS service and must be cut loose.

The simple fact that the FTO is now working with students dictates that things will be different. "Extra" people will now be on the unit. The FTO will be responsible for her own actions and those of her partner, as well as those of the student. Ah, yes . . . the student.

The FTO is certainly an authority figure to the student. The student will be acutely aware of the FTO's power. Possibly even before meeting the FTO, the student may be wondering if the FTO will be mean, hard-nosed, inflexible, or out to trick him into doing something stupid.

FTOs must balance their responsibility to the EMS system and the safety of patients on the one hand and the needs of the student on the other. While maintaining the highest standards of patient care, the FTO will be teaching and evaluating the student and acting as a role model. However, the FTO will not be able to communicate effectively with the student until a basic sense of trust and credibility has been

FTOTips ☑

The FTO should make these concepts clear to the student: "I cannot be your 'best friend'; however, I will be fair, I will be honest, I will follow the rules, and I *will* help you learn."

established. The FTO can build this trust and credibility through the following actions:

- Being consistent
- Being honest
- Giving positive feedback on the student's strengths
- Being objective in feedback, both verbal and written
- Demonstrating skills instead of assuming that students should already know them
- Correcting errors and omissions early
- Being a good listener
- Resisting the temptation to play head games with the student

These are basic concepts of teaching and positive human interaction, and none of them should be new to the FTO. The greatest challenge for many FTOs will be developing a workable approach to teaching that incorporates all of these traits into the daily routine, for every student, every day.

Effective Teaching Strategies: How People Learn

Hierarchy of Needs

Whether age 18 or 80, EMS students are adult learners. The FTO can begin planning for success by considering a few of the more widely accepted concepts that relate to the adult learner.

In 1970, humanist Abraham Maslow described the "hierarchy of needs," which is shown in **Figure 1-1**. Maslow viewed a person's *physical needs* as being at the lowest level and his *spiritual needs* at the highest. The FTO can use the pyramid in

Maslow's Hierarchy of Needs

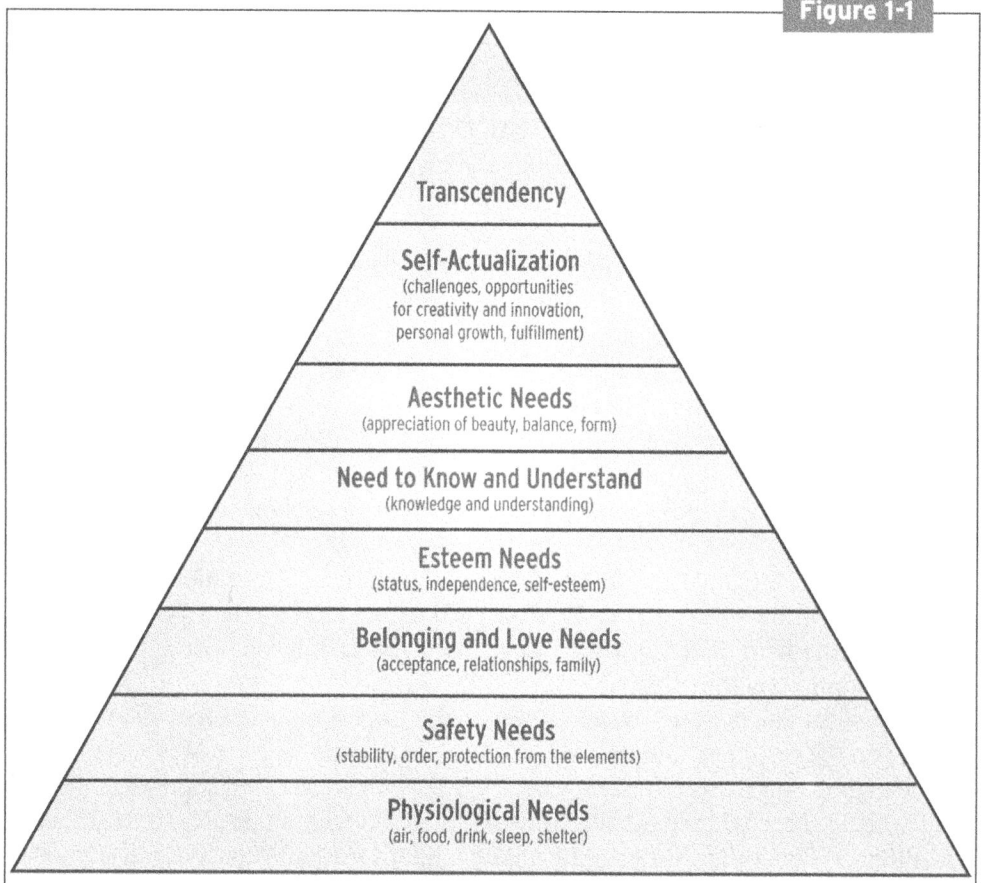

Figure 1-1

Transcendency

Self-Actualization
(challenges, opportunities for creativity and innovation, personal growth, fulfillment)

Aesthetic Needs
(appreciation of beauty, balance, form)

Need to Know and Understand
(knowledge and understanding)

Esteem Needs
(status, independence, self-esteem)

Belonging and Love Needs
(acceptance, relationships, family)

Safety Needs
(stability, order, protection from the elements)

Physiological Needs
(air, food, drink, sleep, shelter)

Figure 1-1 as a blueprint for helping the student achieve success in the field internship.

Individuals strive to fulfill successively higher levels within the pyramid. According to Maslow, an individual will not satisfy higher-level needs unless all the needs below it have been, and remain, satisfied. A wise FTO will take an active role in facilitating the student's efforts to satisfy basic needs so as to facilitate higher-level learning. The faster a student progresses, the less work (guidance) will be required of the FTO. Simple guidance about the location of the coffee pot and restrooms in the EMS station, the location of safety equipment, and introductions to crew members help satisfy some of the student's most basic physiologic needs. It also helps the student begin to satisfy needs related to feelings of safety and belonging.

By anticipating the student's concerns, the FTO can help to minimize them. The FTO can provide answers to some of the questions that are probably flying around in the student's mind, such as:

- "What do I need to do to keep from looking stupid?"
- "Does this FTO grade hard?"
- "What do I do if I disagree with the FTO (I don't want to make her angry)?"
- "How can I please this FTO (and successfully complete the program)?"
- "How can I (at all costs) avoid making mistakes?"

Crafting preemptive answers to questions like these is not hard. The FTO might begin this process by demonstrating that the FTO and student are both members of the same team. Rather than the FTO telling the student what *he* needs to do to succeed, the FTO could start by telling him, "Here's what *we* need to do to get you successfully through the field internship." The FTO serves as a buffer between the student and his new environment. The FTO is the student's guide throughout the field internship journey. A lack of guidance from the FTO will actually create more work for both the student and the FTO. Refer back to Maslow's hierarchy as a model, note that it will take more time for the student to achieve success at higher levels of the pyramid if time is first not invested in satisfying lower-level needs, such as physiologic and emotional needs.

At first, the student may view himself as an outsider who's been inserted into an environment that was already running smoothly without him. The FTO can help put the student at ease in a number of ways. The FTO can brief her partner at the beginning of the day (about her plans for helping the student and the partner's role). The FTO can introduce the student to other EMS providers. The FTO can remind the student that everyone makes mistakes and that she will do her best to keep him from making big mistakes. The FTO answers questions before the student even asks them.

Once the student's more basic needs are met, the FTO can explain the techniques she will use to give instruction. The FTO can explain how she intends to help the student become a successful team leader. With each subsequent patient contact, the FTO will guide the student's performance. As the student's performance improves, he will automatically move on to address higher levels of need fulfillment, developing an increased sense of belonging and self-esteem.

As performance improves, the student will require less guidance from the FTO. The student will be free to focus on fulfilling the need for knowledge and understanding. The FTO will recognize this progress when measurable performance improvement in areas such as decision making, pathophysiology, human behavior, EMS operations, and so forth is observed.

The FTO can address needs related to self-esteem in at least two ways: (1) The FTO can give positive feedback when the student demonstrates successful skill performance and (2) the FTO can make the student understand that there is usually more than one "right way" to perform a task. This gives the student the freedom to perform skills in the ways that are most comfortable to him, based on his life experience. By treating the student as an adult, the FTO has helped him satisfy self-esteem and progress to meeting self-actualization needs.

As the student progresses in the field internship, he becomes more comfortable with the role of team leader and with his place in the EMS team. He can then focus on adjusting the environment to better suit his personal preferences, thereby fulfilling aesthetic and self-actualization needs. The student may find, for example, that he likes to organize his equipment in a certain way. He may prefer to distribute tasks in a certain way (among himself and other providers) during patient care. By accepting the student's approach (as long as it stays within the parameters of acceptable care), the FTO allows the student to find his own niche, and his own style, within EMS. The student is moving ever closer to successful completion of the field internship.

As the student requires less guidance from the FTO, he begins to develop a rhythm as a team leader. He begins to see the value of taking charge and making his own decisions. He will view himself as an increasingly valuable member of the EMS team. He is beginning to understand his place in the larger picture—in EMS, in health care, and in the community at large.

The Art and Science of Helping Adults Learn

The renowned educator Malcolm Knowles first coined the term *andragogy* in 1968, describing it as "the art and science of helping adults learn." He argued that adults learn differently than children do. In contrast with the teaching approach known as *pedagogy*, which many of us experienced when we were children, andragogy makes certain observations about the characteristics of adult learners. **Table 1-1** compares pedagogy and andragogy.

According to Knowles, adult learners are self-motivated. The adult student wants to be involved in the education process. He wants instruction based on discussions and scenarios, rather than on lectures. He wants to have some measure of control—to be an active participant, not an observer. He wants the course content to be applicable to his work ("How will I use this information?"). The FTO can guide the student in a manner that ensures he will be an active participant by

Table 1-1	Assumptions About Participants in the Learning Environment	
	Pedagogy	**Andragogy**
Teacher's role	Giver of knowledge, lecturer	Facilitator, coach
Student's role	Passive learner	Active participant
Motivation	External (I must learn)	Internal (I want to learn)
Course focus	Teacher centered	Student centered
Goals and objectives	Teacher driven	Shared decisions
Purpose of learning	To be used in the future	To be applicable, pertinent now
Student experience	Very little life experience	A wealth of life experience

providing explanations and demonstrations to show the student how to apply his newly acquired knowledge.

The adult learner's prior life experiences affect how the student learns, absorbs, and uses new information; he may need the FTO to give examples that will connect with past experiences (e.g., How many FTOs have used plumbing examples to describe the circulatory system's structure and function?). The adult learner's prior knowledge will affect his or her ability to apply course content and may also determine how much must be unlearned or altered in order for new learning to take place. For example, consider the paramedic student who has several years of experience as an EMT-B.

The FTO can effectively assume the role of facilitator, guide, and coach by prompting the student to take action throughout the course of each patient contact and by providing feedback after the patient contact. This approach forces the student to become an active participant, to make treatment decisions, to act on those decisions, and to contribute to the discussions that follow each patient contact. By acting as a facilitator through prompts and feedback, the FTO becomes more trustworthy in the student's view. The student will discover that the FTO's actions are both dependable and credible.

Before beginning EMS education, each student will have developed a unique view of the world around him—a view that is based on prior life experiences. He will make decisions that are shaped (at least in part) by these same experiences. He wants to learn and to apply knowledge—and to apply it as soon as possible! It is up to the FTO to find the best way to use this life experience. The FTO's job will be much easier if she has the right tools.

FTOs can use the tools found later in this book to help students accomplish their goals. FTOs should take into account that, because of a unique set of life experiences, each student may require a slightly different instructional strategy. One example of a tool that FTOs can use to modify their teaching strategy will be found in Chapter 4, "More Than One Way."

Many factors influence the manner in which an adult learns. Environment, life experiences, and predisposition to certain learning styles will all have an impact. When FTOs consider these factors and anticipate how they can best be addressed, they will be able to modify their instructions to better suit the needs of adult learners.

Let's move on to the tips and techniques!

FTOTips ☑

Take the time to learn about the student's life experiences. Use this information to develop analogies that will facilitate the student's ability to learn.

References

Anderson, J. R. *Cognitive Psychology and Its Implications* (4th ed.). New York: Freeman, 1996.

Grippen, P., Peters, S. *Learning Theory and Learning Outcomes.* Lanham, MD: University Press of America, 1984.

Knowles, M. S. *Andragogy in Action: Applying Modern Principles of Adult Learning.* San Francisco: Jossey-Bass, 1984.

Maslow, A. H. *Motivation and Personality* (2nd ed.). New York: Harper Row, 1970.

Merriam, S., Caffarella, R., Wlodkowski, R., Canton, P. *Adult Learning: Theories, Principles and Applications.* San Francisco: Jossey-Bass, 2003.

Check Your Knowledge

1. The FTO can build trust and credibility by:
   a. Being fair
   b. Being honest
   c. Being objective when giving both verbal and written feedback
   d. All of the above are correct answers

   The correct answer is **d**. Fairness, honesty, and objectivity are all traits that enhance the FTO's credibility with students and coworkers alike.

2. According to Maslow's Hierarchy of Needs, a student will need to fulfill all _____ level needs before attempting to fulfill needs at a _____ level.
   a. Higher, lower
   b. Lower, higher
   c. The order in which a student fulfills needs does not impact learning

   The correct answer is **b**. According to Maslow, an individual cannot fulfill higher level needs until needs at lower levels have been satisfied, and continue to be satisfied.

3. According to Knowles, adult learners:
   a. Are not self-motivated
   b. Want to be active participants in learning
   c. Do not want the course content to be applicable to their work
   d. All of the above are correct answers

   The correct answer is **b**. Adult learners want to be active participants. They are also self-motivated, and they *do* want course content to be applicable to their work.

4. According to Knowles, adult learners:
   a. Require constant motivation from the FTO
   b. Want to be active participants in learning
   c. Want the course content to be applicable to his or her work
   d. Only **b** and **c** are correct answers

   The correct answer is **d**. The adult learner is *self*-motivated. The adult learner wants to be an active participant in the learning process. The adult learner also wants course content to be applicable to their work.

5. Assume that your student has the following needs: 1) Making friends at the station, 2) Viewing himself as a competent EMS provider, and 3) Acquiring adequate clothing for cold weather. Using Maslow's Hierarchy as a reference, place the needs in the order in which the student will be mostly like most likely to address them:
   a. 1, then 2, and then 3
   b. 2, then 3, and then 1
   c. 3, then 2, and then 1
   d. 3, then 1, and then 2

   The correct answer is **d**. According to Maslow; the student will not be able to satisfy more complicated needs until the more basic needs have been met.

6. If Malcom Knowles were a field training officer, he would most likely describe his role as that of:
   a. Facilitator and coach
   b. Lecturer and giver of knowledge
   c. Facilitator and giver of knowledge
   d. Provider of teacher-centered instruction

The correct answer is **a**. Knowles contends that adult learners are self-motivated and that student-centered instruction will be most effective. Adult learners are likely to progress more quickly when encouraged to be active participants and contribute to decision making. For these reasons, the FTO is likely to be most effective when acting as the student's facilitator and coach.

2 Structure of the Field Internship

KEY POINTS

- Established rules and expectations make the field internship more effective.
- FTO roles and responsibilities should be included in the rules governing field internships.
- The field internship is divided into three phases: observation, instruction, and evaluation.
- During the observation phase, FTOs demonstrate effective team leadership.
- During the instruction phase, students learn how to be team leaders.
- During the evaluation phase, students succeed or fail based on performance as team leader.

The ultimate evaluation of student performance occurs during the field internship. FTOs understand that students have demonstrated their didactic skills by passing written exams and by knowing how to defibrillate manikins in the school's laboratory. FTOs also hope that students have learned how to assess vital signs on patients in the emergency department. However, FTOs, course coordinators, and future employers *all* want to know if these students will be able to assess and treat patients in the field environment when the pressure is really on. Everyone's questions will be answered if students are required to complete an effective and successful field internship.

No two EMS systems' field internships will be exactly the same. This chapter provides a simple template that can be applied to any system's field internship. Issues such as call volume, system finances, and local performance standards will ultimately determine the amount of time that each system is able to set aside for field internships.

Some EMS systems use a full-time internship that occurs at the end of the education process, whereas others use a part-time internship that runs throughout it. Some systems use a combination of part-time and full-time internships. The three phases of field internship described in this chapter—observation, instruction, and evaluation—can be applied to any field internship format.

Rules

Roles and responsibilities for both students and FTOs should be defined within the EMS agency's rulebook. The rulebook establishes goals and objectives for students, as well as for FTOs. Throughout this text, the rulebook will be referred to as the *manual* (i.e., manual for students and FTOs). An existing manual (*Manual for Paramedic*

Students and Instructors) can be found in Appendix A. This manual has been included as an example of how one might be prepared.

The manual should explain the expected length of the field internship and define what each student must accomplish in order to successfully complete each phase. The manual should also describe the roles and responsibilities of the FTO. One example of an FTO responsibility is the manner in which student performance will be documented. The FTO's documentation will be a key element in determining whether a student has met the criteria for successful completion of the field internship.

Students demonstrate proficiency by performing a wide variety of EMS-related skills. FTOs help students learn how to perform each of these skills. The ultimate goal is for the student to learn how to provide adequate medical care to each patient encountered. FTOs are not likely to encounter many students who hit the ground running and become competent providers within a week or two. At the beginning of the field internship, it is much more likely that the FTO will have to guide the student, step-by-step, throughout the performance of many basic skills. Within this book, the FTO's guidance is referred to as "prompting." How and why an FTO uses prompts will be explained in subsequent chapters.

Prompts are only mentioned here because they are also used as tools for measuring and trending student progress. Students generally require fewer and fewer prompts (i.e., less help from the FTO) as they gain experience and confidence. This measurable decrease in the number of prompts acts as a trending signal to the program director as well as to the FTO and the student. A decrease in the number of prompts indicates that a student is ready to enter the final stage of the field internship. What follows is a basic template for a field internship.

Observation Phase

The first phase of the field internship is *observation*. The FTO serves as the team leader during this phase. The FTO assumes the role of "student," demonstrating what the student will be required to do as the team leader in the instruction phase. The student is expected to closely observe the FTO's demonstrations of how things should be done.

During this phase, the FTO explains *what* is being done and *why* it needs to be done. The FTO also answers any questions the student may have. The FTO is demonstrating how to be an effective team leader. The student is observing the FTO to see how an experienced provider performs her duties. The student watches as the FTO makes decisions, utilizes resources, performs psychomotor skills, multitasks, and demonstrates good affective behavior. The student also performs any tasks assigned by the FTO. Performance of tasks (such as taking vital signs or starting an IV) will help the student begin to feel like a member of the EMS team.

Many tasks assigned to the student (e.g., initial assessment, intravenous access) will have time limits. These skills must be performed without exceeding the time limits for performance to be considered satisfactory. These time limits introduce the student to the fast pace that is necessary in the provision of effective patient care. In the observation phase, the student gets the opportunity to experience this fast pace without having the overall responsibility for managing patient care. The observation phase also gives the student the opportunity to perform skills that may have, until now, only been practiced in the lab or in hospital settings.

FTOTips ☑

Every EMS agency needs to have a "rulebook" that defines the roles and responsibilities for both students and FTOs.

The observation phase typically lasts for a minimum of two shifts (e.g., an 8-hour shift, a 12-hour shift), but can extend as long as a week or two. Time allotted to the observation phase generally depends on the call volume. The student needs to have an adequate opportunity to watch the FTO demonstrate the team-leader role.

Instruction Phase

During the instruction phase, the student serves as the team leader, assuming responsibility for managing all aspects of patient care. The FTO guides the student through each patient contact by correcting any student errors. These corrections are made in the form of real-time prompts from the FTO. Each of these prompts should be documented by the FTO. The student receives a pass-fail score for each patient contact. As described later in the text, these scores can be determined by simply counting the number of prompts given by the FTO.

The student is required to manage a minimum number of patients in order to successfully complete the instruction phase. Students may also be required to achieve a minimum overall percent success rate (e.g., a 60% success rate) in order to complete the instruction phase successfully. Patient contacts can also be separated into categories based on the severity of a patient's injury or illness. For example: Priority 1 = immediate threat to life or limb; Priority 2 = potential threat to life or limb; Priority 3 = does not require immediate EMS intervention at this time.

Some systems require a student to manage a minimum number of high-acuity patient contacts (e.g., of the 25 patients the student must manage, at least 20 must have a high acuity, that is, Priority 1 or 2). Students often have more difficulty managing high-acuity patients. Establishing a minimum number of high-acuity cases ensures that a student does not move to the evaluation phase without demonstrating the ability to handle unstable patients.

An upper limit should be set on the amount of a time a student can spend in the instruction phase. The length of this phase will depend on call volume and, possibly, on the acuity of the patients the student encounters. Care should be taken not to shorten this phase even if numerical criteria are met; *the student gains experience through time served in the field environment as well as through the number of patient contacts.*

Recall that FTOs assign pass-fail grades based on the number of prompts a student has received on each patient contact. A patient contact will be assigned an unsatisfactory grade if the student has received too many prompts. The student is responsible for learning from prompts the FTO has given. Prompts can be tracked by type to see if the student is making repeated errors.

Similar prompts that are given repeatedly are called *repetitive prompts*. For example, say a student has been prompted three times in two days to apply oxygen to patients who are obviously short of breath. Assume that the student is allowed three repeated prompts. Starting with the fourth repetitive prompt, the student would receive a failing score for each similar prompt that occurs. This scoring technique holds the student accountable, and the student must demonstrate that he can learn from his mistakes. Repetitive prompting can have a serious impact on the student's overall success rate. Repetitive prompts should be tracked throughout the course of the field internship.

In many systems, students periodically meet with the field internship coordinator. This gives the coordinator a chance to review the FTO's documentation with the student. This is also a logical time for the student to receive a progress assessment. Areas for improvement can be identified and success rates calculated. Trends can be noted (i.e., progress, no progress, regression). The coordinator can opt to give the student a written progress report that details trends that have been noted.

Periodic evaluations should include action plans the student can use to improve performance. These action plans are often directed at student performances that required repetitive prompting from the FTO. The coordinator can discuss the written evaluation and answer any questions the student may have. The coordinator and student can also review the student's evaluation of the FTO's performance.

Many EMS systems expect each of their FTOs to apply the rules from the manual in the same way. The coordinator should use student feedback to evaluate the performance of the system's FTOs.

Once the minimum criteria for *successful* completion of the instruction phase have been met, the student will move on to the evaluation phase of the field internship.

FTOTips ☑

Action plans spell out in clear terms exactly what the student needs to do to improve his performance.

Evaluation Phase

The evaluation phase is the final phase of the field internship. Some systems allot the same amount of time to both the instruction phase and the evaluation phase. The student continues to operate as the team leader during this phase. The FTO continues to observe, assist, and document the student's performance. The bar for demonstration of successful performance is set a little higher during the evaluation phase. For example, a system that allows three prompts (per patient contact) during the instruction phase may allow only one prompt during the evaluation phase. Students would then be assigned a failing score if they receive more than one prompt per patient contact during the evaluation phase.

The FTO continues to prompt the student whenever necessary. Hopefully, the student will continue to learn during the evaluation phase. Within a system that counts prompts, students receive failing grades whenever they require too much prompting. No matter what format, or the number of allowable prompts, the FTO is trying to back away from the student during the evaluation phase.

The FTO has been the student's safety net throughout the course of the internship. That safety net will no longer be available once the student completes the evaluation phase. Students need to demonstrate that they can provide patient care that is safe, timely, appropriate, and within local protocol, and that such care can be provided without too much help from the FTO.

As in the instruction phase, the student may be required to team-lead a minimum number of patient contacts in order to complete the evaluation phase. The system may require a higher percent success rate (e.g., 75%) for satisfactory patient contacts. A requirement for a minimum number of high acuity patients may also be implemented.

The program coordinator should continue to provide verbal and written feedback to the student. As in the instruction phase, performance evaluation is based on documentation provided by the FTO. The student successfully completes the field internship by satisfying the criteria established in the manual. However, what happens if a student is having difficulty meeting the criteria for successful completion of the field internship?

Remediation

Many types of remediation can be made available to students participating in a field internship. Remediation is an integral, continuous, and ongoing component of the instructional methods described in this book. The FTO uses prompts to remediate unacceptable student performance. For example, "Take vital signs now," "Listen to lung sounds now," and "Pull traction here while you are starting this IV" are all prompts that can signify unacceptable performance.

Prompts serve as immediate real-time remediation. They ensure the delivery of timely and appropriate patient care. They also ensure that the student has the opportunity to learn *how* and *when* a certain skill should be performed. The FTO does not attempt to "fix it later." The FTO remediates by immediately correcting any student error or omission. However, another form of remediation could occasionally be utilized. The second form of remediation should not be required very often.

Say that a student is having difficulty with only one or two skills. Perhaps the student has difficulty performing initial assessments within the allotted time. Maybe the student has been unable to consistently obtain complete medical histories from the patients.

The second form of remediation is usually defined by either a specific period of time (e.g., two shifts, one week) or a specific number of satisfactory performances (e.g., 10 initial assessments at a success rate of 90% or greater). The student would generally be responsible for targeted skills (initial assessments, medical histories) during this period of remediation. All other responsibilities are assigned to other members of the EMS team. This format removes the pressure of multitasking and team leadership from the student's shoulders and allows the student to concentrate on improving performance for the targeted skills.

Unfortunately, the student, while enjoying the relative comfort and safety of a remediation period, could run out of time. The student could discover that there is so little time remaining (after completing remediation) that it is impossible to meet the criteria for successful completion of the field internship. For this reason, students often choose to avoid this type of remediation.

Check Your Knowledge

1. During the observation phase of the field internship, students should:
   a. Observe as the FTO demonstrates team leadership skills
   b. Perform certain skills at the direction of the FTO
   c. Both a and b are correct answers

The correct answer is **c**. Although it is important for the FTO to demonstrate team leadership skills, the FTO assigns certain skills to the student in order to make him feel more like a member of the EMS team.

2. During the instruction phase of the field internship, students should be evaluated on their ability to function as a team leader.
   a. True
   b. False

The correct answer is **a**. Following the observation phase, the student will always be evaluated based on his performance as team leader.

3. An upper limit should be set for the amount of time a student is allowed to stay in the instruction phase of the field internship.
   a. True
   b. False

The correct answer is **a**. Some students will ultimately be unable to complete the field internship. Those students who are unable to meet the criteria for successful completion of the instruction phase within the allotted time frame should not be permitted to continue the field internship portion of their program.

4. A(n) _____ plan spells out in clear terms what a student needs to do to improve his performance.
   a. Care
   b. Quality improvement
   c. Action
   d. Collaboration

The correct answer is **c**. FTOs use action plans to map out a plan the student can use to improve his performance.

5. During the evaluation phase of the field internship, students are generally permitted _____ prompts (per satisfactory patient contact) than they can have during a satisfactory patient contact within the instruction phase.
   a. More
   b. The same amount of
   c. Fewer

The correct answer is **c**. Students should be permitted fewer prompts during the evaluation phase since fewer prompts are required for students who are demonstrating improvement in the team leadership skills.

3

Four Questions: A Self-Test for the Field Training Officer

KEY POINTS

- FTOs perform a self-test by asking four questions.
- Self-test questions remind FTOs that student performance does not have to be perfect.
- An FTO self-tests to determine why "something just doesn't seem right."
- Additional questions may help explain why something isn't right.

Occasionally, an FTO will get the feeling that "something just doesn't seem right." FTOs may get this kind of feeling when they have made a mistake. A mistake has been made whenever the student receives the wrong grade. An FTO's credibility decreases when a student receives the wrong grade. An FTO can use the self-test presented in this chapter to eliminate errors in documentation.

This chapter gives FTOs a simple method for double-checking their documentation. This chapter also provides a method FTOs can use to decide why something "just doesn't seem right."

The self-test can be used to address a number of the FTO's doubts, such as:
- Was the student's performance acceptable?
- Did I give the student the wrong grade?
- If I graded the student's performance incorrectly, where did I go wrong?

Putting the Cart Before the Horse

Shouldn't the FTO learn how to grade student performance before learning how to conduct a self-test? For a number of reasons, the answer is no. The self-test questions help an FTO develop a feel for what performance is acceptable and what performance is unacceptable. The self-test questions provide FTOs with an easy method for dealing with new situations. FTOs will also use the questions to figure out why something just does not seem right. In most situations, however, FTOs will not need to use a self-test.

In most cases, student performance is easy to evaluate. Each FTO is an experienced provider who is comfortable performing a wide range of skills. Most FTOs understand what needs to be done in almost any situation. They also know how quickly these tasks need to be accomplished. In most instances, it will be easy for an FTO to determine if a student's performance is satisfactory or unsatisfactory. FTOs will only need to use the self-test questions if they get that nagging feeling that something just isn't right.

Something Just Isn't Right

The FTO has instructed the student, evaluated the student's performance as an EMS team leader, and assigned scores that seemed to be consistent with the student's performance. The FTO isn't certain that something is wrong, but something just doesn't seem right.

The FTO begins to wonder: "Did I give the student a grade that was too low?" "Did I give too high a grade?" Or, "Is this feeling related to something other than the student's grade?" The FTO can use the following questions to figure out what is causing this funny feeling.

Question 1: Were the Student's Actions Safe?

The first question, "Were the student's actions safe?" is easy to answer. The FTO would have corrected the student if the student's actions had placed anyone at risk. For example, an FTO would not let a student give a patient the wrong medication. The student would be prompted to apply oxygen if the patient was having trouble breathing. An FTO would not let a student step across a high-voltage electric wire at the scene of a motor vehicle crash.

In such instances, the FTO can simply conduct a mental review of the patient contact. The FTO asks, "Was there anything I had to correct so that nobody would be at risk of injury?" The student's actions were unacceptable if the FTO had to provide a prompt to keep the student from doing something that was not safe (e.g., "Oh yes, I had to remind him to put gloves on."). The FTO moves on to the second question if this question was answered in the affirmative: "Yes, the student's actions were safe."

> **FTOTips** ☑
>
> Student performance should be graded as unacceptable if the FTO steps in to prevent the student from taking action that would jeopardize the patient.

Question 2: Were the Student's Actions Timely?

The second question, "Were the student's actions timely?" can also be answered without too much difficulty. A student's actions were timely unless the FTO had to take one of the following actions: Did the FTO have to intervene by performing a skill that was supposed to be the student's responsibility? Did the FTO have to prompt the student to move faster because a skill performance was taking too much time?

Once again, the FTO conducts a mental review of the patient contact. The FTO asks, "Did I have to intervene?" and "Did I have to prompt the student to go faster?" The student's actions were not timely if the FTO had to intervene or prompt the student to go faster. The FTO can move on to the third question if the answer to this question was affirmative: "Yes, the student's actions were timely."

Question 3: Were the Student's Actions Appropriate?

The third question, "Were the student's actions appropriate?" is sometimes easy to answer, but not always. A student will occasionally say or do something that is inappropriate. The FTO may have had to tell the patient, "He (the student) didn't really mean to say that" or, "He didn't really mean to do that." The FTO can be reasonably certain that the student's actions were inappropriate whenever it is necessary to apologize.

It does not matter whether an FTO had to apologize to the patient, to the family, or to other providers. There is no acceptable excuse for poor behavior. Most students are on their best behavior when they are with an FTO. If the student displays poor affective behavior when with the FTO, what will that student do when the FTO is not around? An FTO must address any problem related to affective behavior. Inappropriate behaviors should result in the student receiving an unsatisfactory score for that patient contact.

If the student's action is an obvious example of poor behavior, why would an FTO ever doubt that the student received the correct score? An FTO might get the feeling that something just doesn't seem right because the inappropriate behavior did not occur during a patient contact. This is an interesting situation. A student may demonstrate good behavior throughout the course of most patient contacts, but may not behave well between calls. This type of situation is likely to give the FTO an uneasy feeling.

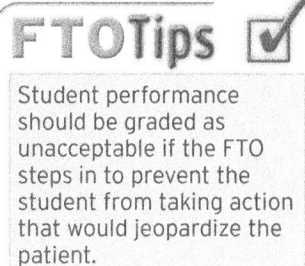

In this type of situation, the FTO is uneasy for a very good reason. The FTO may have worked with people who had similar behavior problems. These are often the providers who frequently arrive late to begin a shift. They don't perform their share of station duties. They are rude to their coworkers. Even though they usually stop short of blatantly bad behavior in public, these providers find a way to irritate patients, family members, and coworkers on a somewhat regular basis.

An FTO should document every incident of unacceptable student behavior. This is why the FTO should ask, "Were the student's actions appropriate?" The FTO must document a student's inappropriate behavior anytime this question is answered in the negative. The FTO moves on to the fourth question whenever the answer is "Yes, the student's behavior was appropriate."

Question 4: Were the Student's Actions Within Local Protocol?

The fourth question, "Were the student's actions within local protocol?" is also usually easy to answer. FTOs are very familiar with the local standard of care. A student's actions were probably within protocol if the FTO did not have to intervene. The student's actions may not have been within protocol if the FTO did have to intervene. The FTO mentally reviews the patient contact by asking: "Did I have to intervene because the student went outside of protocol?" The FTO grades the student's performance in accordance with the answer to this self-test question.

This completes the four-question self-test. Answers to the self-test questions will guide FTOs through the student evaluation process. However, what does an FTO do when an uneasy feeling persists, even after the four questions have been answered?

Two More Questions

Occasionally an FTO will continue to feel that something isn't right even after asking the four self-test questions. The FTO gave the student instruction. The FTO evaluated how well the student performed during each patient contact. The student has received satisfactory scores for most patient contacts. It appears that the student is progressing nicely.

Assume that the FTO still had some nagging doubts. The self-test questions could be used to determine if the student's actions were safe, timely, appropriate, and within local protocol.

The FTO used the self-test to recheck the validity of her grading. Say the FTO answered all four questions with a "Yes" and still has that nagging feeling! The FTO has one more self-test that can be used.

This self-test begins with an assumption. The FTO says, "Let's assume this student graduates and begins working in my EMS system." The FTO then asks two more questions:

- Would I be comfortable if this student were called to care for a member of my family?
- Would I be comfortable working with this student if he were assigned as my regular partner?

Why would an FTO even consider asking these two questions? This student seems to be providing patient care that is safe, timely, appropriate, and within local protocol. Why would an FTO continue to have that gut feeling that something just isn't right?

The First Reason

The FTO may not have evaluated some of the student's patient contacts correctly. This happens when a student is not held to the performance standards described in the manual. The FTO may have made mistakes. It happens. The FTO was reluctant to give the student bad scores and made too many allowances. The authors' experience indicates that allowances are most frequently made in the following areas:

- The student's ability to make good decisions during a patient contact
- The student's ability to make an accurate differential diagnosis
- The student's ability to demonstrate acceptable affective behavior

Whenever an FTO's uneasy feeling lingers, these two questions can be used as the final self-test. If the answer to the first question is "No," the FTO should go back and take a closer look at the four-question self-test. That nagging feeling that something just isn't right is probably related to the student's ability to provide patient care. The FTO needs to double-check to make sure the student's actions really were safe, timely, appropriate, and within local protocol.

The four self-test questions address issues that relate directly to patient care. FTOs use these questions to determine which part of the student's patient care was inappropriate. But what if an FTO's feeling is not directly related to a patient care issue? The FTO might have to look for another reason that something just isn't right.

The Second Reason

If the answer to the first question is "Yes," then the FTO's concern is probably not a patient care issue. The FTO now wants to know the answer to the second question, "If this student is assigned as my regular partner, will I be comfortable working with him?"

The FTO can relax if the answer is "Yes." The uneasy feeling is probably unfounded. But what if the answer is "No"? The FTO now has to take a closer look at certain student behaviors. The FTO needs to look closely at behaviors that might make the student a poor prospect for employment. These behaviors can be overlooked by FTOs when they do not have a direct impact on patient care or when the program has no mechanism for measuring the behaviors. Some educational programs may have few mechanisms for measuring certain student behaviors such as tardiness, dress code violations, poor personal hygiene, poor interpersonal skills with coworkers, or failure to perform routine tasks such as station duties or equipment checklists.

These two additional questions are a reminder to FTOs. They remind FTOs to continue evaluating student performance, even when the student is not actively involved in patient care. An FTO will continue to feel that something isn't right if instances of poor behavior, such as those listed above, are not addressed.

The Other Side of the Coin

Sometimes an FTO feels that something just isn't right when a student receives a failing grade. Once again, the FTO can self-test by asking the four self-test questions and, if necessary, the two additional questions.

If an FTO answers all self-test questions with a "Yes," the student probably received failing grades that were not warranted. This typically occurs when an FTO requires the student to meet too high a standard. The FTO may have used a personal standard instead of relying on the guidelines described in the manual for students and FTOs.

Students occasionally receive failing grades resulting from a different kind of FTO error. Sometimes an FTO may not agree with a student's method for performing a skill. This might happen when a student performs a skill in a manner that is new to the FTO. FTOs need to remember that there may be more than one "right" way to perform that skill.

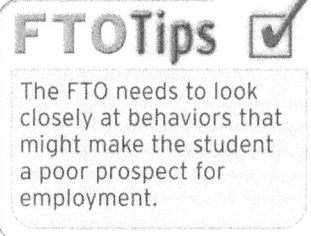

FTOTips ☑
The FTO needs to look closely at behaviors that might make the student a poor prospect for employment.

Check Your Knowledge

1. The student should receive an unsatisfactory score for any patient contact where his performance was _____.
   a. Not timely
   b. Not appropriate
   c. Not within local protocols
   d. All of the above

The correct answer is **d**. The student's performance as a team leader was not acceptable if the FTO had to prompt for safety, speed, or inappropriate behavior, or to correct student actions that were outside the limits of the local standard of patient care.

2. The student's performance is likely to be unacceptable if the FTO would not want to _____.
   a. Work with this student if he successfully completes the field internship
   b. Have this student be responsible for care of the FTO's family member
   c. Both a and b are correct answers

The correct answer is **c**. The student's overall performance as an EMS team leader is most likely unacceptable if one, or both, of these situations exist.

3. At what point should an FTO begin documenting unacceptable behaviors?
   a. Immediately after the first incident of unacceptable behavior
   b. After the FTO has warned the student about this behavior once
   c. After the FTO has warned the student about this behavior twice
   d. Only after patient care is jeopardized

The correct answer is **a**. Each individual incident of unacceptable behavior should be documented at the FTO's earliest convenience. There should be no occasion where an incidence of unacceptable behavior is not documented.

4. In which situation would an FTO be most likely to make allowances for an unacceptable student performance?
   a. The amount of time required to establish intravenous access
   b. The amount of time required to perform an endotracheal intubation
   c. The amount of time required to control arterial bleeding
   d. The student's inability to make an accurate differential diagnosis

The correct answer is **d**. Virtually every student will eventually be able to learn how to perform physical skills correctly, and in a timely fashion. Unfortunately, a certain percentage of students will be unable to make an accurate differential diagnosis when placed in a time-critical environment such as the field internship.

More Than One Way

4

KEY POINTS

- Any skill can usually be performed in more than one correct way.
- FTOs must avoid the "my way or the highway" syndrome.

This chapter explains why it is important for FTOs to keep an open mind. Unnecessary problems occur when an FTO says to the student, "Just do it my way." This approach requires the student to perform each skill without deviating from the FTO's preferred method.

The FTO should avoid single-minded styles of instruction and evaluation. Instruction and evaluation will be more effective if an FTO focuses only on whether a skill performance was acceptable. How closely a student's skill performance matches that of the FTO should not be the determining factor.

FTOs Are Human

FTOs want to find an easy way to evaluate student performance. What is the simplest way for an FTO to evaluate a student's performance? It is when the student is required to perform a skill in *exactly* the same way the FTO would perform that skill.

A student who does not perform the task just as the FTO does must be doing something wrong. Or is he? Unfortunately, this style of evaluation is all too common. Many FTOs fall into the do-it-my-way trap when they first begin to teach. Is this style of instruction and evaluation really wrong?

Consider an example. Say that the FTO is left-handed, and the student is right-handed. Should an FTO make the student use his left hand to start an IV because that's how the FTO does it? Obviously, the answer is no. This example might appear to be a little extreme, but it does make a point.

Every provider is unique. Techniques for performing skills vary from person to person. FTOs should not penalize a student based solely on differences in technique. How could an FTO change her approach to evaluating student performance? The FTO can ask, "Is the student's technique getting the job done?" "Was the skill performed at the right time?" and "Were there any safety issues that made the student's performance unacceptable?"

For example, say the student applies a splint using a technique the FTO has never seen before. The question is "Was it effective?" Assume that it *was* effective. The splint adequately immobilized the limb without compromising motor, sensory, or circulatory function. Does it matter that the FTO has never seen it done like that before? In a sense, the answer is both yes and no.

No, It Doesn't Matter

The answer is "no" because the purpose of the splint is to immobilize the injured extremity. The splinting technique is acceptable when it fulfills the criteria for skill performance. The technique needs only to be safe and to not delay patient care.

Yes, It Does Matter

The answer is also "yes" because an FTO may learn something by observing the student's technique. The FTO can mentally file this technique away for future use. The FTO may show this technique to another student who has been having difficulty using the standard technique.

It is easy for FTOs to recognize whether a student's techniques are similar to their own. An FTO's job becomes more difficult when it is acknowledged that there may be more than one way to correctly perform a skill.

What process should FTOs use when evaluating techniques they have never seen before? The FTO can run through a mental checklist (critical performance sheet) while the student is performing a skill. The FTO should only intervene if the skill performance is *not* safe, is *not* timely, is *not* appropriate, or is *not* within the standard of care.

This sounds like extra work, but FTOs make this extra effort because it is likely to produce better long-term results and because this is ultimately the FTO's responsibility. Student performance improves at a more rapid pace when students are able to perform skills using the techniques that fit them best.

Consider the following example. Say that the FTO's unit is dispatched to a call for a patient who is having difficulty breathing. The student has determined that the patient requires placement of an oral airway and ventilatory support with a bag-mask device and oxygen. The student inserted an airway adjunct and began ventilating the patient. This student has very small hands. The student used both hands to get a seal with the mask and then compressed the bag by squeezing it between his forearm and thigh. Chest rise and fall indicated that each ventilation was providing an adequate volume of oxygen.

The FTO had never used this technique and had never seen it performed in this way. What should the FTO do? The FTO might think that this technique looks ugly. Does it matter if it's not a picture-perfect technique? The FTO evaluates the student by using the four-question self-test. Were the student's actions safe, timely, appropriate, and within the standard of care?

The FTO watches the student apply the bag-mask device, observing to see if chest rise and fall appears to be adequate. The FTO looks for color change in the patient's skin and auscultates for presence of lung sounds with ventilations. The FTO completes a mental checklist on the skill performance. The FTO will intervene only if the student's actions are not safe, timely, appropriate, or within protocol. The FTO will not interrupt the patient contact unless there is risk to the patient or the provider.

The FTO will not have to intervene as long as the student is getting the job done. The FTO may elect to discuss this ventilation technique after this patient contact is complete. The FTO can use this discussion to see if there is a better method for the student to use and to find out how many methods the student has already tried. The FTO can ask, "What happened when you tried those other methods?"

FTOTips ☑
Do not interrupt a student's skill performance just because it is different from your technique. Interrupt the student's performance only when it is unsafe, too slow, inappropriate, or outside the local standard of care.

FTOTips ☑
The student might perform a skill in a way that is safe, timely, appropriate, and within the standard of care—even though the technique is nothing the FTO has ever seen before.

FTOTips ☑
By allowing the student to perform a task in an unusual way, the FTO's agency can be strengthened. How, you ask? Let's assume for a moment that the FTO's regular partner has difficulty with the bag-mask device because her hands are small. After she sees the student's technique, she gives it a try, and it works for her, too. Her skills have improved, as well as her confidence.

The FTO will have earned the student's trust by not imposing the my-way-or-the-highway method of evaluation during the course of the patient contact. The FTO may even have learned a new technique that can be passed along to the next student that has small hands.

However, situations will occur that require the immediate attention of the FTO. These are situations where the student's actions are *not* safe, timely, appropriate, or within local protocol. What should the FTO do when a situation like this occurs?

The FTO will give the student a "prompt"!

Check Your Knowledge

1. The student's performance is likely to suffer if the FTO forces the student to perform each skill "just like the FTO does it. . . ."
   a. True
   b. False

   The correct answer is **a**. A student's performance will improve at a more rapid rate if he is allowed to use techniques that are the best "fit" for him.

2. The student's development as a team leader may be slowed if he is allowed to use techniques the FTO is not familiar with.
   a. True
   b. False

   The correct answer is **b**. To the contrary; unnecessary interruptions by the FTO are more likely to destroy the student's confidence, thereby slowing his progress as team leader.

3. The student is performing c-spine stabilization on a supine patient during a patient contact. During the process of securing the patient to the long backboard, the student reaches for one of the head blocks, and holds the head with his knees. The FTO should:
   a. Immediately correct the student's action, and later document the correction
   b. Observe the performance and ask the student about his technique during debriefing
   c. Note that the patient's head was being held securely by the student's knees, and ask about the technique later
   d. Correct the student's action immediately, and ask about the technique during debriefing.

   The correct answer is **c** *or* **d**. If the goal is to control movement of the head, and the head is being held safely with the knees, the FTO may choose to do nothing but observe and discuss later (Is there any text or course that allows this type of c-spine stabilization? Yes. Consider c-spine control during intubation of the trauma patient. Some trauma courses consider use of the knees an acceptable option.). If the FTO is uncomfortable allowing the student to continue with this technique during the patient contact, she may choose to direct the student to hold the head with both hands, apply the head block herself, and review the technique during debriefing. If the student can demonstrate and support that the technique is acceptable, then there should be no documented prompt (however, the FTO should document the discussion).

Prompting the Student

KEY POINTS

- Prompts motivate students to take action.
- Prompts may be either verbal or physical.
- Physical prompts are less disruptive to the flow of a patient contact.
- Verbal prompts are more effective when posed as a question.
- Preset time limits tell the FTO when to give a prompt.
- Learning opportunities are lost if the FTO prompts too quickly.
- Late prompts from the FTO delay patient care.

This chapter contains tips and techniques for giving prompts to students. The two basic types of prompts are verbal prompts and physical prompts. This chapter explains the role of prompting in instruction and evaluation, explaining *why* a prompt is given, *how* a prompt could be given, and *when* a prompt should be given. This chapter provides techniques that FTOs can use to streamline their current methods for prompting students.

What Is a Prompt?

What exactly is a prompt?

- **As an adjective:** Something is *prompt* when it is punctual or done without delay. Prompts motivate the student to perform each skill at the right time (done at once).
- **As a verb:** *Prompt* means (to the FTO) to help out or to suggest. The FTO may use a prompt to help the student perform a skill correctly. The FTO may use a prompt to suggest a better method for performing a skill.
- **As a noun:** A *prompt* is an action taken by the FTO to improve the student's performance, ensure his safety, and enhance patient care.

Prompts are either physical or verbal.

Physical Prompts

A *physical prompt* is any type of nonverbal prompt. A raised eyebrow can be a prompt. A nudge from the FTO's elbow can be a prompt. Most physical prompts will be given as hand signals from the FTO.

The FTO might use a cupped hand to prompt the student to apply a nonrebreather mask. The FTO might hold a hand up in the universal stop sign to prevent the student from performing a skill incorrectly. The FTO might place the fingers of one hand on the wrist of the other arm to indicate that it's time for the student to take a pulse (**Figure 5-1**).

Many FTOs trained in this method of instruction have been using these types of

> **FTOTips** ☑
>
> Prompts are the most important of the FTO's tools. The FTO will use prompts to make the student act or to correct an action. These prompts will ensure that patient care is always safe, timely, appropriate, and within the local standard of care parameters.

Examples of physical prompts.

Figure 5-1

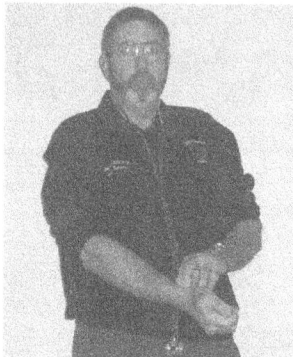

(A) Check pulse.

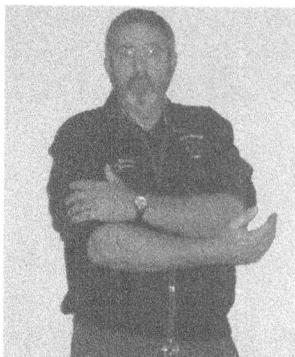

(B) Check blood pressure.

(C) Provide supplemental oxygen.

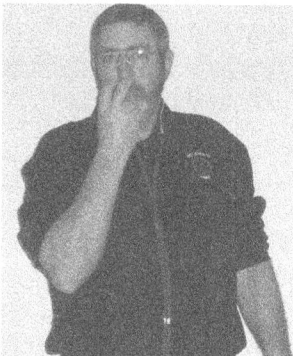

(D) Insert nasal cannula.

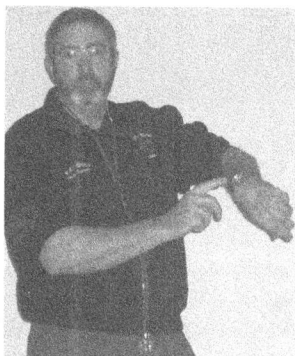

(E) We need to move faster.

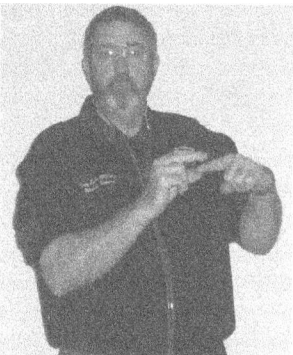

(F) Use pulse oximeter.

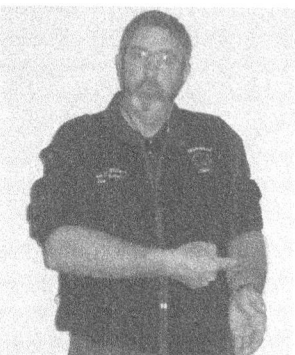

(G) Provide IV fluids.

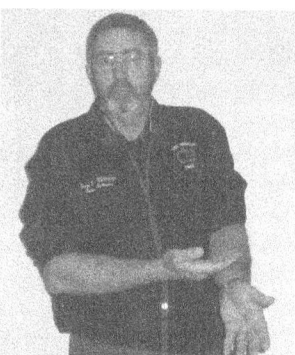

(H) Check patient's skin condition.

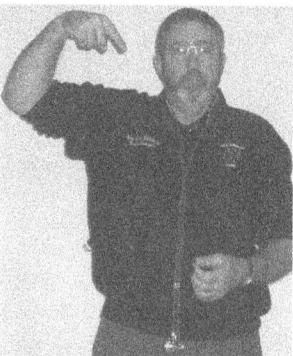

(I) Take a look around (finger drawing a horizontal circle).

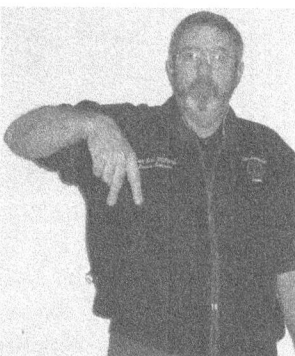

(J) We need to roll.

prompts for a long time. What are the benefits of physical prompts? Wouldn't it be easier for the FTO to just tell the student what to do?

The advantages of physical prompts include the following:

- **Physical prompts are silent.** The FTO can give a physical prompt without interrupting the flow of student-patient communication.
- **Physical prompts can be given from behind the patient.** The prompt will be outside of the patient's line of sight and (once again) will not interrupt student-patient communication.

The FTO can use physical prompts to unobtrusively guide the student through the patient contact. The patient will not hear or see these prompts. The patient will focus on the student and will not be distracted by the FTO's prompts.

The student is in charge of the patient contact and will be evaluated based on his performance as the team leader. What would likely happen if the FTO gave all prompts as verbal directives? For example, "Put the patient on oxygen now," "Ask if she has any allergies," or "Get vital signs now." The patient would quickly lose confidence in the student if the FTO were to give too many verbal prompts. The student would then have difficulty maintaining control of the patient contact. The student is trying to learn how to be a team leader. The student is not likely to perform effectively as a team leader if the patient believes the FTO is controlling the patient contact. It will be easier for the student to maintain control if the FTO uses unobtrusive physical prompts.

Physical prompts do not destroy the patient rapport that the student is working hard to develop. Physical prompts are excellent tools. They make it possible for the FTO to guide the student through each patient contact without attracting the patient's attention. But what should the FTO do if a physical prompt is not working or if a physical prompt is not appropriate for a certain situation?

Verbal Prompts

Sometimes the FTO will have to use a verbal prompt. The following are examples of when verbal prompts are appropriate:

- **Physical prompts may not work when things are moving too quickly.** If the student is about to do something that could harm the patient, the FTO will have to step in and say "Stop" or "Why don't we try this."
- **Some prompts cannot be given physically.** For example, it is often difficult to use a physical prompt to get the student to ask a question about the patient's medical history.
- **Physical prompts may not be effective when the FTO needs to know what the student is thinking.** The FTO wants to make sure the student is headed in the right direction. In this case, the FTO may have to ask, "What protocol are you going to use for this patient?"

Is there a right way to give verbal prompts? In most cases, there probably is a right way. The critical questions are:

- Which kinds of verbal prompts are the best tools for an FTO?
- Which types of verbal prompts are most effective?

Most EMS providers work in teams. Partners talk to each other all the time. Think about what style of verbal communication works best between partners. Do partners give directives to each other? For example, "You start the IV! I'll give the medications!" Or, is it more likely that help is solicited by asking questions? For example, "Can you start the IV while I get the medications ready?"

Most people are more receptive if they are *asked* to do something and less receptive when they are *ordered* to do something. This is true for the FTO's partner. It also is true for the patient, and it certainly is true for the student. The FTO should

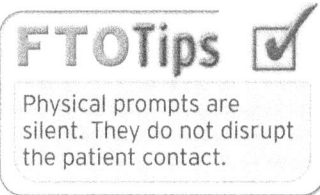

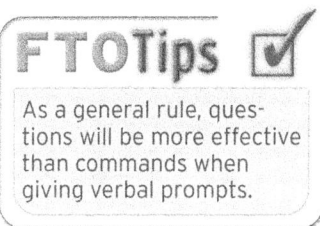

FTOTips ☑

Physical prompts are silent. They do not disrupt the patient contact.

FTOTips ☑

As a general rule, questions will be more effective than commands when giving verbal prompts.

consider everyone's point of view when getting ready to give a prompt. Compare the following two styles of giving verbal prompts to the student:

- The FTO could say, "Put the patient on oxygen" (directive). Or, the FTO could say, "How much oxygen did you want to apply?" (question).
- The FTO could say, "Take the patient's pulse" (directive). Or, the FTO could say, "What did you get for a pulse rate?" (question).

It is likely that both the student and the patient will be more comfortable with prompts that are phrased as questions. The patient will think that the FTO is simply asking the student for a piece of information. The student will understand that the FTO is really prompting the student to apply oxygen or to count the pulse rate. The rapport between patient and student, however, will not be disrupted when the FTO uses a question to give a prompt.

Inadvertent Prompts

The FTO does not have control over everything that happens during a patient contact. The student may become "clued in" when another provider begins to take action or when another provider makes an offhand comment. These clues are referred to as *inadvertent prompts*. They might come from a family member (e.g., "He has diabetes."). They might come from the patient (e.g., "Can you give me some oxygen?"). However, most inadvertent prompts come from other providers.

Consider the following example. The FTO's partner opens the airway bag in preparation for oxygen administration. The FTO is not supposed to prompt until 30 seconds have elapsed. The FTO has been waiting for the elapsed time to reach 30 seconds, but the student sees what the partner is doing and puts the patient on 4 liters via nasal cannula.

The FTO should document each inadvertent prompt. The FTO can make a decision later as to whether to include such prompts in the scoring process. The FTO can make this decision when completing the critique form for the patient contact. The FTO's options with regard to documenting inadvertent prompts will be explained in more detail within the chapters on scoring.

▨ Why Does the FTO Use Prompts?

The FTO wants certain things to happen when the student receives a prompt. The FTO uses prompts to guide the student through each patient contact. It is the responsibility of the FTO to ensure the following:

- The student performs each skill safely.
- The student performs each skill within an appropriate time frame.
- The student behaves in an appropriate manner.
- The student provides patient care that is consistent with local protocols.
- The patient receives acceptable patient care.

This involves a lot of hard work on the part of the FTO. In many instances, it would be easier for the FTO to just go ahead and perform the skill. The FTO invests the extra effort so that the student can learn how and when to perform each skill. The student will learn more quickly if the FTO is adept at giving prompts.

Prompts are the most essential tool for guiding a student through the instruction and evaluation phases. Prompts serve many purposes:

- Prompts can be used to improve skill performance.
- Prompts can be used to ensure that each skill is performed at the appropriate time.
- Prompts can be used to ensure that each skill is performed safely.

FTOTips ☑

The FTO should become adept at using prompts. Effective prompting will allow students to learn at a faster pace (putting the pieces of the puzzle together more quickly).

- Prompts can be used to ensure that patient care is performed in accordance with local protocol.
- Prompts can be documented, creating a record of student performance and FTO instruction.
- The number of prompts given can be used to determine a score for a patient contact.
- The number of prompts given can be used to trend student performance.

Let's look at how prompts are used to address each of the preceding items.

Prompts Used to Improve Skill Performance

Say that the student is having difficulty locating the radial pulse during the initial assessment. The FTO can simply say, "It's there. It's fast, regular, and normal in strength. Move on to checking the skin" (for color, moisture, and temperature).

The FTO saves time using this approach. Unfortunately, the student does not learn how to properly locate the pulse when the FTO takes this approach. It is likely that the FTO will have to deal with this same issue over and over again until the student learns (without prompts) how to locate the pulse quickly.

Instead, the FTO can use the situation as an opportunity to teach the student how to locate the radial pulse. For example, the FTO could say (and demonstrate), "Sometimes it is hard to find the pulse. Locate the knob at the distal end of the radius. Use light pressure with your index and middle fingers. Palpate medially, adjacent to this knob, and slowly move up (proximally) the forearm until you locate the pulse."

In this case, the FTO invests a small amount of time teaching the student how to locate a radial pulse. This investment will be repaid many times over the course of other patient contacts. This student will probably not require repeated prompts on how to find the pulse. The student will also gain confidence in his ability to assess patients.

Prompts Used to Ensure That Skills Are Performed at the Appropriate Time

Say that the student is performing an initial assessment. The student notes that the patient is short of breath, is breathing fast, and has retractions. The student then begins to assess the patient's circulation.

At this point, the FTO moves into the student's line of sight and offers the physical prompt for the application of a nonrebreather mask (cupped hand in front of face). The student can either apply the nonrebreather mask or, better yet, delegate that skill to another provider while continuing the initial assessment.

The FTO used this prompt to ensure that oxygen was applied in a timely manner. The FTO's prompt gave the student an opportunity to make the connection between the assessment of labored breathing (rapid respiratory rate and retractions) and timely therapy (oxygen applied via nonrebreather mask). This student was given the opportunity to learn that oxygen should be applied quickly when a patient exhibits signs of respiratory distress.

Prompts Used to Ensure That Skills Are Performed Safely

Consider a situation in which the student has located a laceration on the patient's left thigh and has noted that it is bleeding freely. The student opens a package of sterile 4″ × 4″ gauze and makes a move to apply the dressing material. The FTO says, "Do you want me to apply those 4 × 4's while you put gloves on?"

In this situation, the FTO used a verbal prompt to make sure that the student did not suffer a potential exposure to a communicable disease. The FTO also used this prompt to teach the student a safer method for performing this particular skill.

The FTO gave the prompt in the form of a question. The FTO used an unobtrusive prompt so that the student could maintain control of the patient contact.

Prompts Used to Ensure That Patient Care Is in Accordance with Local Protocol

Say that the patient was ejected from a motorcycle while traveling at a high rate of speed. The patient had a large abrasion and contusion on his forehead. The student determined that the patient was breathing at a slow rate, but had adequate ventilations. The student also found that the pulse was slow but very strong.

The student found an obvious deformity to the left leg during the rapid trauma assessment. Pedal pulses were present in both feet. The student called for a lower-leg splint to be applied before loading the patient in the ambulance. Local protocol requires trauma patients to be removed from the scene as quickly as possible. The FTO asked, "Could we save time by using the backboard to splint the leg until we get the patient into the ambulance?"

The FTO used a question to prompt the student to see if the student could make a more appropriate decision. The FTO wanted to see if the student understood the protocols for trauma patients and could decide which skills must should be done on scene and which skills should be done en route to the hospital.

The student responded by saying, "That would be good. Let's immobilize the patient on the backboard and then we'll move him to the unit. Joe (the FTO's partner) can finish splinting the leg while I continue the assessing the patient on the way to the hospital."

In this scenario, the patient received care that was consistent with local protocols and the student had the opportunity to learn how to make a more appropriate decision at a trauma scene.

Prompts Are Documented

Consider the following example. The patient is a 52-year-old male presenting with altered mental status. Trauma was ruled out, and oxygen was applied to the patient. The student asked the spouse if the patient has any "medical problems." The spouse indicated that the patient has no medical problems.

The FTO prompted by asking the spouse a specific question: "Is your husband an insulin-dependent diabetic?" The spouse responded: "Oh yes, he takes insulin, but he's never had any medical problems since he started taking it."

In this scenario, the student had the opportunity to learn the value of asking more specific types of pertinent negative history questions. The FTO demonstrated an efficient method of asking history questions that can be useful for patients with altered mental status.

The FTO will document this prompt (pertinent negative question for insulin-dependent diabetes) on a critique form. The specific procedure for recording this documentation will be discussed in later chapters.

Each documented prompt serves two purposes. First, the FTO documents the prompt so that the student will be reminded to ask specific pertinent negative questions. Second, the FTO will count the total number of prompts that occurred during that patient contact. The FTO will then assign a score to each patient contact. This score will be determined by the total number of prompts a student received.

Prompts Determine the Student's Overall Score for Each Patient Contact

For the following example, assume that the student is in the instructional phase of the field internship. The FTO prompted the student once in the initial assessment competency (to apply oxygen). The FTO prompted the student once in the history

---

FTOTips ☑

Each prompt serves at least two purposes. A prompt first serves to motivate the student, guiding the student to provide more appropriate care to the patient. Each prompt also serves as a tool for evaluating student performance, since every prompt will be documented on a critique form.

competency (to ask about allergies). The FTO prompted once in the physical exam competency (to check lung sounds).

Each of these prompts was documented on the critique form for that particular patient contact. The student's school allows the student to be prompted as many as three times and still receive a satisfactory overall score during the instruction phase. The student would receive a satisfactory overall score for this patient contact because no more than three prompts were received.

However, the student might be allowed only one prompt (per patient contact) during the evaluation phase. If this student received the same three prompts during the evaluation phase, the student would receive an unsatisfactory overall score because more than one prompt was given.

These are just two simple examples of how prompts can be used to score patient contacts. The reader will be offered a number of more detailed descriptions for scoring patient contacts in later chapters.

Prompts Measure Trends in Student Performance

The FTO documents every prompt given to a student. These prompts are recorded on critique forms. The program coordinator can track the number and types of prompts to determine whether a student's performance is improving. Consider the following two examples:

- The student needed two to five prompts on every patient contact during a two-week period. There was no trend of improvement.
- The student received two to five prompts on every patient contact during the first week of the internship. In the second week, the student received one to three prompts on every patient contact. This represents a measurable trend of improvement.

The FTO will generally be required to provide fewer prompts as the student gains more experience. Trending the number of prompts provides measurable data that indicates whether a student is making progress.

When to Prompt

Prompts serve as the cornerstone for the method of instruction and evaluation presented in this book. Many examples of how an FTO might prompt a student will be presented in subsequent chapters. But *when* exactly should the FTO give a prompt?

Limits for Elapsed Times

Is it likely that the student and FTO will agree on what is an acceptable speed for performing a skill? How will the FTO know when the student is taking too much time? Is it possible to have a standard that tells the FTO how much time is too much time? How can this standard for acceptable speed be consistently applied from one FTO to another?

Questions like these can make a person's head spin. These questions apply to FTOs and students alike. Everyone can benefit if there is an easily understood system for determining how much time is too little or too much.

The student will not be able to meet the FTO's expectations if the FTO does not allow enough time for the student to perform a skill. However, patient care might be delayed if the FTO allows too much time. The bottom line is that time limits must be reasonable. Additionally, the FTO must have an accurate method for measuring elapsed time. Time limits will not be effective if any one of these criteria is not met.

Tools for Tracking Elapsed Time

The student and the FTO are in this battle together. Both are dependent on the FTO's ability to track elapsed time. The FTO needs to have a tool that measures the speed of the student's skill performance. The FTO's watch is that tool.

Every FTO should have a watch. Is there anything else the FTO will need? The FTO should have two other tools. The first is a set of established time limits for the performance of certain skills. The second is a technique the FTO can use to measure the amount of elapsed time. FTOs use this technique to reset their internal clocks. FTOs rein in their internal clocks by making a habit of checking their watches (elapsed time) just as they have made a habit of checking their mirrors while driving. Listed below are some examples for elapsed time limits. These elapsed time limits are based on a decade of trial and error in the field, feedback from many FTOs, and direct observation of student performance. *The reader should not consider these times to be absolutes, but rather recommendations.* They are simply a list of time limits that have proven to be effective within one statewide EMS system.

Sample Limits for Elapsed Time

Initial Assessment: 30 Seconds

The FTO begins tracking elapsed time when the student first has physical contact with the patient (**Figure 5-2**). Elapsed time ends when student has verbalized findings for the entire initial assessment (i.e., c-spine, airway, breathing, circulation, disability, exposure as necessary).

Initial Interventions: 30 Seconds

Elapsed time begins when the student notes a deficit (e.g., obstructed airway, fast respirations, absent radial pulses). The student is required to address each deficit within 30 seconds of the time the deficit is noted. An exception is made for a patient with a compromised airway. Only 15 seconds may elapse before the student must be prompted to open an obstructed airway using a manual technique. Elapsed time ends when the student acts (or delegates actions) to address the deficit (e.g., applies oral airway, applies oxygen therapy, initiates chest compressions).

Application of Protocol or Standard of Care: 3 Minutes

Elapsed time begins with the first physical contact between student and patient. Elapsed time ends when the student verbalizes the selection of a protocol and begins to implement the appropriate treatment regimen.

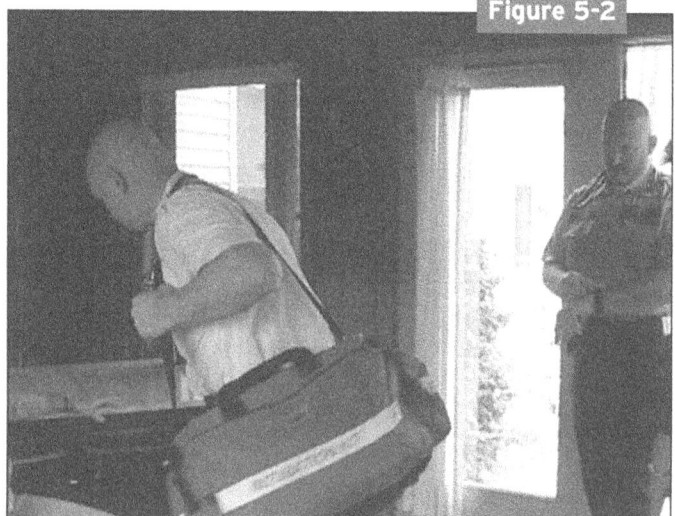

FTOTips ☑

The reader might ask if it is really feasible for the FTO to check her watch during a patient contact. It is not only feasible, but it is also an enormously effective tool. Periodically tracking elapsed time will remind the FTO to give students enough time to think and act. And ... it will also remind the FTO exactly when it is time to give a prompt. An FTO that relies on personal intuition and experience (for timing prompts) is simply applying their own personal standards to the student's performance evaluations.

The FTO checks his watch at the start of the patient contact.

Figure 5-2

Reassess: 5 Minutes for a Stable Patient or 30 Seconds When the Patient's Condition Is Deteriorating

Elapsed time begins with the completion of initial assessment and initial interventions. Elapsed time ends at 5 minutes when the patient's condition remains stable. The student is required to reassess the patient within 30 seconds whenever there is a precipitous change in the patient's condition.

Change of Therapy: 30 Seconds

The student may be required to change the course of the patient's treatment. This situation most often occurs when the patient's condition worsens quickly. The student should be given no more than 30 seconds to initiate the appropriate therapy whenever reassessment of the patient indicates a change of therapy is required. The student should be prompted to take action once elapsed time has reached 30 seconds.

Intravenous Access: 3 Minutes

Elapsed time begins with application of the tourniquet. Elapsed time ends when the line has been secured and is running at the correct flow rate. The student should receive an unsatisfactory score for the IV skill if the time limit is exceeded.

Tracheal Intubation: 1 Minute

Elapsed time begins when the blade first enters the oral cavity. Elapsed time ends when the tube has been inserted into the trachea and all required verification techniques have been used to confirm placement. The student should receive an unsatisfactory score for the skill if the time limit is exceeded.

Exceptions

The FTO can overrule the limits for elapsed time. The FTO may elect to give a prompt before the time limit has been reached. The FTO is most likely to do this when a patient requires an immediate intervention. In addition, the FTO may extend the time limits whenever extenuating circumstances make it impossible for the student to complete a skill within the stated time limits. The FTO is the student's teacher and evaluator. The FTO will be the best judge of how much time is too much, or too little, in any set of circumstances. FTOs just need to make sure they have their internal clocks under control.

The FTO's Internal Clock

Preset limits for elapsed time give FTOs a reason to slow down their internal clocks. Once FTOs have a reason to slow down, they can concentrate on the mechanics for keeping their clocks under control.

An FTO's internal clock runs faster than a student's internal clock. FTOs process information faster and make decisions more quickly than students do. FTOs act more quickly once a decision has been made. Students are not able to think or act as rapidly as FTOs do.

Time limits remind FTOs to slow down their internal clocks. FTOs should show restraint to give the student the opportunity to learn and demonstrate proficiency. However, FTOs should not slow down so much that patient care is delayed. FTOs should prompt students to take action whenever the preestablished time limit for a skill has been reached.

This system benefits everyone involved. Patients receive timely care. Students know in advance (from reading the manual) exactly how much time has been allotted to performing a particular skill. FTOs know they do not need to prompt students until the time limit has been reached.

Teaching Points

Occasionally, an FTO will jump the gun and give the student a prompt before the time limit has been met. What should the FTO do now?

Sometimes the FTO will be unable to resist temptation and will offer a prompt before the student has exceeded the limit for elapsed time. Is this student going to complain? Certainly! The FTO probably felt giving the prompt was in the patient's best interest. A prompt that comes too early will not be counted against the student because the FTO did not follow the rules for elapsed time. Prompts are documented as teaching points whenever this type of situation occurs. The FTO documents the prompt and marks it with a "TP" (teaching point). The FTO does not include the teaching point when counting the number of prompts for scoring purposes.

The FTO's Partner

Occasionally, the FTO's partner jumps the gun. This is likely to occur when the student is not moving fast enough to suit the partner. The partner's internal clock has not been adjusted; the partner's clock is moving just as fast as ever.

The FTO should offer the partner an explanation of how the limits for elapsed time work, letting the partner know that the student will not be allowed to pitch a tent in the patient's living room. The partner is more likely to slow down if the limits for elapsed time are explained.

Using a Stopwatch

FTOs can make their lives simpler by wearing a stopwatch (or a wristwatch with a stopwatch function). Time passes quickly during patient contacts, making it easy for FTOs to lose track of time. A simple remedy is for FTOs to use stopwatches. Then the FTO just pushes a button at the beginning of each skill performance and a glance at the watch will tell how much time has elapsed.

Many FTOs elect to start the stopwatch when the student first makes contact with the patient. They track elapsed time by periodically checking the watch. FTOs will develop a rhythm for tracking time by glancing at their watches. This will keep their internal clocks from running too quickly.

The FTO will not have to estimate elapsed time once after periodically checking for the amount of time that has elapsed. The FTO will know exactly when to prompt because the amount of time that has elapsed has been checked periodically.

Most FTOs take notes throughout the course of a patient contact. Some FTOs make a note of the time when the student first contacts the patient and then continue to track how long it takes for the student to perform certain skills. FTOs can also record elapsed time ("prompt O_2 at 30 sec") whenever a prompt is given for a particular a skill. These notes will be very helpful when it is time for the FTO to document the student's performance.

FTOs should practice glancing at their watches, tracking how much time has elapsed. Eventually, the FTO will develop a good rhythm for tracking time by periodically glancing at the stopwatch. It would be reasonable to check the stopwatch every 30 to 60 seconds.

1. The FTO used two curved fingers to prompt the student to apply oxygen via nasal cannula. This is an example of a _____ prompt.
   a. verbal
   b. physical

   The correct answer is **b**. Showing the student two curved fingers is a physical prompt. The FTO did not have to speak (verbalize) to the student.

2. The FTO asked the patient if he was an insulin-dependent diabetic. This is an example of a _____ prompt.
   a. verbal
   b. physical

   The correct answer is **a**. The FTO gave a prompt by asking the question about insulin dependence.

3. The FTO's partner opened the oxygen bag before the FTO was ready to prompt. The student then asked the partner to apply oxygen to the patient. This is an example of a(n) _____ prompt.
   a. physical
   b. verbal
   c. inadvertent

   The correct answer is **c**. The FTO did not give the student a prompt. The student was prompted to take action when he saw the FTO's partner open the oxygen bag. This type of prompt is called an inadvertent prompt.

4. The FTO gave a prompt before the amount of elapsed time had been exceeded. This prompt is considered a(n) _____.
   a. physical prompt
   b. verbal prompt
   c. inadvertent prompt
   d. teaching point

   The correct answer is **d**. A prompt is considered a teaching point whenever the FTO gives a prompt before the student has exceeded the time limit. Teaching points are documented so that the student can learn from the FTO's written comments. Teaching points are not counted as prompts when the FTO is scoring the patient contact.

6 Student Verbalization

KEY POINTS

- Students verbalize assessment findings to the FTO.
- Students verbalize treatment decisions to the FTO.
- Verbalization ensures that the student is not doing the right thing for the wrong reason.
- Students verbalize effectively by simply talking to the patient.

The method of instruction and evaluation presented in this book requires the student to verbalize frequently. This chapter describes the process of verbalization and explains why it is important. Specifically this chapter addresses: (1) why the student is required to verbalize; (2) what may go wrong if the student does not verbalize; and (3) the most effective methods for verbalizing. This chapter discusses how and when a student should verbalize.

Why the FTO Requires the Student to Verbalize

The FTO requires the student to verbalize for a number of reasons:

- The only way for the FTO to be sure the student has completed an accurate assessment is for the student to verbalize the assessment findings to the FTO.
- The FTO needs to know if the student has selected the most appropriate course of treatment. The student must verbalize the treatment plan to the FTO.
- The FTO needs to know if the student recognizes a change in the patient's condition. The student verbalizes any changes to the FTO and explains the course of action.

These are just a few of the many good reasons why FTOs require students to verbalize. The FTO needs to know what the student has seen and heard. The FTO must know exactly what the student intends to do in any given situation.

Time passes quickly during a patient contact. The FTO must be prepared to prompt the student whenever the student should take action. The FTO must be prepared to correct a student's mistakes. What happens if the FTO waits too long for the student to verbalize? Any delay in prompting is likely to delay the delivery of patient care. The FTO may hesitate because it looks like the student is heading in the right direction. Many FTOs may believe they can read their students' minds, but they should not assume they know what their students are thinking.

Let's look at one example. Say that the student does the right thing for the wrong reason. The FTO watches the student lean over a 68-year-old patient. The patient is on a bed in the hallway of an extended-care facility. The patient is pale and cool to the touch. The student reaches over to take a radial pulse on the right arm. The FTO is unable to detect a radial pulse while checking the left arm. The registered nurse is giving a report to the student. The nurse says that the patient has had severe abdominal pain for 12 hours. The nurse also says that the patient has emesis that is the color of coffee grounds. The student looks at the FTO and states, "We need to leave now."

The FTO believes the student has recognized signs of shock. The FTO interprets the student's statement as recognition that the patient needs to get to a definitive care facility quickly. However, the student is *actually* thinking, "We're not going to get any good information from this nurse, and I want to get out of this facility because it smells terrible in here."

This student has misled the FTO by doing the right thing for the wrong reasons. What can the FTO do in a situation like this? The FTO can simply respond with the question "why" after the student says we need to leave now. Hopefully, the student will be wise enough not to voice his opinions in front of the nurse; but if he does . . . the FTO will know immediately that this student is not likely to become a useful EMS provider.

The FTO will, however, find the needed information by prompting the student to verbalize. The patient should ultimately benefit from the student's verbalization. Additionally, the FTO will gain important information from the student's verbalization. Verbalization helps speed the process of caring for the patient. Verbalized information helps the FTO decide whether or not to prompt the student.

Verbalization Is Beneficial to the Student

The student verbalizes to make sure that the FTO does not overlook any skills that have been performed.

The FTO will be busy during every patient contact. It is not unusual to have several conversations taking place at the same time during a patient contact. All providers (student, partner, FTO) may be busy performing tasks while the following conversations are taking place:

- Providers are talking to each other about who is going to do what task.
- Providers are relaying information to each other about the patient's signs and symptoms.
- The student is gathering history from the patient.
- The partner is gathering additional history from family members or bystanders.

The FTO may not hear everything that the student says. The FTO may not see the student perform a particular skill. The student does not want the FTO to overlook a task that has been performed. It is the student's responsibility to communicate with the FTO, thereby ensuring that an aspect of skill performances is not overlooked.

What Happens When the Student Does Not Verbalize?

The FTO will be forced to make assumptions if the student does not verbalize. The FTO will have to assume the following:

- **History questions were not asked** (if the FTO did not hear the student ask the questions).
- **Physical exam procedures were not performed** (if the student does not verbalize what was done).
- **Results of exam procedures were not valid** (if the student does not verbalize the correct results).
- **Delegation of tasks was not done** (if the FTO did not hear the student delegate).
- **No protocol was selected** (if the student did not verbalize the treatment plan).

It is the student's responsibility to verbalize. It is the FTO's responsibility to explain why verbalization is important. The student is not likely to be successful if he or she does not communicate fully with the FTO.

The FTO will occasionally fail to hear or see a skill the student has performed. The student will say, "I did that (skill)." In this situation, the FTO will most often ask the partner to verify whether the student actually performed the skill. The FTO should assume the student has not performed a skill whenever that performance cannot be verified by the FTO's partner.

Student Verbalization Scenarios

Scenario 1

The student approaches the 63-year-old patient. He says to the patient, "You don't have to speak. It may be easier for you to answer by nodding yes or no. Are you having trouble breathing?"

The FTO will love this verbalization because it indicates that the student has already recognized signs of respiratory distress. The student is not required to repeat the question (and answer) for the FTO. The student can simply look at the FTO. The FTO will give a prearranged signal (a thumbs-up will work) to tell the student that the FTO heard the exchange between the student and the patient.

The student then continues through the initial assessment. He says to the FTO, "The airway is patent. Breathing is fast and labored. Retractions are present." The student tells the patient, "My partner is going to give you oxygen through a mask." He finishes the assessment by reporting, "The pulse is fast, regular, and strong. The skin is pale, moist, and warm. There is no bleeding."

This student has demonstrated the ability to accurately complete an initial assessment and to address the noted deficiency in breathing.

This may seem like verbalization overkill, but there are reasons for doing it this way. The FTO needs to know if the student can (1) find the deficit in breathing and (2) make an immediate decision to apply oxygen.

What should the FTO do if the student verbalizes a deficit in breathing and moves on to the assessment of circulation without addressing the deficit? The FTO must be prepared to prompt immediately. The FTO should move into the student's line of sight and show him a cupped hand to the face as a prompt to apply oxygen via a nonrebreather mask.

Would it make any difference if the student was not required to verbalize? If verbalization was not required, when would the FTO know to offer a prompt? The FTO can wait to see if the student is going to take action, then wait a little longer, and then a little longer. What are the likely results of this style of instruction?

The following could occur if the FTO waits too long before supplying a prompt:

- Patient care may be delayed.
- The student may not learn to associate certain signs and symptoms with a specific course of treatment. For example:
  - Are there signs and symptoms of respiratory distress?
  - If so, apply oxygen now!
- The FTO may never know if the student can correctly perform a particular skill. The FTO will have to perform the skill if too much time has been spent waiting to see what the student is going to do. The FTO will not know if the student observed the following:
  - Was the student seeing what the FTO was seeing (retractions)?
  - Was the student hearing what the FTO was hearing (wheezes)?
  - Was the student planning to perform the correct treatment in a timely manner (oxygen)?

Scenario 2

The student and FTO are listening to lung sounds simultaneously. The student reports, "The bases are decreased and there are wheezes in all other fields."

What should the FTO do if these assessment findings are accurate?

- Nod "yes" or give a thumbs-up.
- Say "OK."

If these findings are not accurate, the FTO will need to give a prompt. The student's verbalization might give the FTO important information. The FTO now knows that the student did not identify rhonchi. She can use this situation as an opportunity to teach. The FTO could say, "Let's listen again. Listen at this spot. That coarse sound is rhonchi."

Scenario 3

The student is assessing the patient's pulse rate. The FTO is confirming the results on the other arm. The pulse rate on the pulse oximetry monitor is displayed as 66 per minute. The student reports that the pulse rate is: "66."

The good news is that the student verbalized his findings. The bad news is that the FTO believes the student may have just read the pulse rate off of the monitor. The FTO asks, "How did you get that rate?" The following are some possible student responses:

- "Let me check again" (or "OK, you got me!").
  - The FTO has caught the student being dishonest.
- "I counted 33 beats in 30 seconds and multiplied by 2" (that will work!).
  - This is probably an accurate finding.
- "I counted 16 beats in 15 seconds and multiplied by 4" (this doesn't work).
  - This student needs to work on his multiplication skills.

The student's verbalization will give the FTO a lot of information. Something as simple as a verbalized pulse rate can become a valuable tool. The FTO will find that there are many uses for this tool.

As noted earlier, the FTO can use verbalization to learn if the student's behavior is appropriate. The student who said "Let me check again" is venturing into dangerous territory. Students must be honest. Students must be accountable for their actions. The FTO will want to keep a close rein on the student who said "Let me check again." This FTO would be wise to document the student's reply ("Let me check again"), verbatim, on the critique form.

Scenario 4

The patient is the restrained driver of a motor vehicle that crashed while traveling at a moderate to high rate of speed. There is no entrapment. The patient has an open femur fracture. The patient is not alert. The airway is patent. Breathing is rapid and nonlabored. Radial pulses are absent. The skin is pale, moist, and cool.

Assume that local protocol dictates that trauma patients be transported within 10 minutes if there are no extenuating circumstances. Also assume that students are expected to verbalize their protocol selection (plan of action) within 3 minutes. Three minutes have elapsed since the student first contacted the patient. Oxygen has been applied. The initial assessment and rapid trauma assessments have been completed.

The FTO gives a prompt by asking the student, "What's your plan?" The student responds, "This is a high priority trauma patient. I want to continue c-spine precautions and do a rapid extrication. We need to get this patient flat on the board because he has no radial pulses. We need to be off scene in less than 10 minutes. We'll finish the assessment and treatment while we are on the way to the trauma facility."

This student has given the FTO a lot of good information. The FTO now knows what the student plans to do. The FTO can give additional prompts if they are needed or simply okay the student's plan of action if it is appropriate.

This verbalization would probably take less than 30 seconds of the student's time. This is time well spent.

Notice that the student did not report every finding. This is acceptable. Time is a very valuable commodity; it should not be wasted. The on-scene FTO will be the best judge of exactly what information needs to be verbalized.

This FTO is probably assuming that the student has not yet verbalized all of his findings. The FTO will wait until the unit is on the way to the hospital. Then, if the student does not verbalize, the FTO will prompt him to speak. The FTO needs to know if the student can fill in the gaps (e.g., blood sugar, vital signs, lung sounds, history information).

FTOTips ☑

Having the student verbalize by talking directly to the patient is a powerful tool for the FTO. Whenever the student is verbalizing to the patient, several good things are happening. The first is that the student sounds more like a team leader. The second is that the patient will be fully informed about what the EMS team is doing. The third is exactly what the FTO needs: She is hearing all assessment findings, all history questions, and all plans for treating the patient. Armed with this information, she will know precisely when a prompt is needed.

Scenario 5

This student is ready to verbalize his initial assessment findings using a more efficient method of verbalization. He is going to verbalize by talking directly to the patient. The patient is a 64-year-old male. The patient's spouse says that he has a history of chronic obstructive pulmonary disease. An albuterol inhaler is on the table in front of the patient.

The student introduces himself and says to the patient, "You look like you are having trouble breathing." The patient confirms this finding. The student continues, "Your airway is OK, but you are breathing fast and you have some muscle retractions, which means you are working hard. I'm going to give you oxygen through a mask. Your pulse is a little fast but it is strong and regular. Your skin is a little pale and moist but it is warm. You don't seem to be bleeding anywhere."

The student has not spoken directly to the FTO. He reported his findings to the patient. He established a rapport with the patient by telling the patient what he was finding and what he intends to do for the patient.

The FTO can give a sign (e.g., a thumbs-up) to indicate that she has heard the student's findings. The FTO will give a prompt only if the student needs guidance.

Scenario 6

The student takes the blood pressure of his 57-year-old patient. He says to the patient, "Your blood pressure seems to be a little high. It's 148 over 82. Is that about normal for you?"

The FTO has heard the student's blood pressure findings. The student will not be required to verbalize the blood pressure directly to the FTO. The patient remains the focus of the student's attention. The FTO will only give a prompt if the student's blood pressure findings are inaccurate.

Scenario 7

The patient is a 50-year-old male who was stung by a bee. His chief complaint is shortness of breath. He is alert during the initial assessment. He presents with hives and audible wheezing. Oxygen was applied and transport was initiated. The patient suddenly became pale and diaphoretic. He began to complain that he was nauseous and dizzy.

The student immediately said to the patient, "You may be having an anaphylactic reaction. Your pulse is weaker than before. We are going to lower your head just a little bit to help with the dizziness. We are also going to recheck your blood pressure and lung sounds now."

The student verbalized that he recognized a change in patient condition and that he is taking appropriate actions to care for the patient. Once again, the student verbalized by speaking directly to the patient. The student will not be required to repeat this conversation directly to the FTO. The patient remains the focus of the student's attention. The FTO will give a prompt only if it becomes necessary.

Scenario 8

Let's continue with the patient from the preceding example. The patient became dizzy and nauseous. His blood pressure dropped to 70/50. He became severely short of breath, and the pulse oximeter would not produce a valid reading. Local protocol dictates that the EMT-B can assist the patient with administration of an epinephrine auto-injector for patients in anaphylactic shock.

The patient had initially indicated that he had an epinephrine pen in his pocket. The patient's level of consciousness has deteriorated to the point where he now responds only to physical stimulus.

The EMT-B student gently shakes the patient and advises him, "Sir! We are going to help you with the injection now. We are going to clean a site on your thigh. That's where we will give the injection." From this statement, the FTO knows what the student intends to do. The patient remains the focus of the student's attention, and the FTO will prompt only if it is necessary.

Students verbalize to keep the FTO informed. They report assessment findings. They report their treatment plan. The FTO uses this information to make decisions about whether to give a prompt. The FTO will not have to prompt the student as long as the student is headed in the right direction.

Check Your Knowledge

1. The student has not verbalized a pulse rate. The FTO must assume that the student has not yet taken the patient's pulse.
   a. True
   b. False

   The correct answer is **a**. The student is responsible for verbalizing the results of his physical examination. The FTO must assume the exam was not completed when the student does not verbalize exam results.

2. The student is required to verbalize his assessment findings (pulse rate, blood pressure, lung sounds, etc.). He can verbalize these findings by including them in his conversation with the patient.
   a. True
   b. False

   The correct answer is **a**. The student can verbalize exam results by including them in his conversation with the patient. This approach keeps the patient's attention focused on the student rather than the FTO.

3. The FTO may occasionally fail to witness (hear or see) a student's skill performance (e.g., vital signs, lung sounds, etc.). The FTO's partner can confirm whether a skill was performed satisfactorily.
   a. True
   b. False

   The correct answer is **a**. The FTO's partner, or any other provider, can confirm whether the student has performed a skill.

4. The student has reported a pulse rate of 89 beats per minute. The cardiac monitor was displaying a pulse rate of 89 when the FTO prompted the student to report a pulse rate. The FTO must assume the following.
   a. The pulse rate is accurate.
   b. The student has made a math error.
   c. The student counted the pulse for a full minute.
   d. The FTO needs to ask the student how he determined the pulse rate to be 89.

   The correct answer is **d**. It is unlikely that the student counted the patient's pulse for an entire minute. The FTO must assume the student read the pulse rate off of the cardiac monitor. The FTO needs to know (1) how the student got that exam result and (2) what the student's behavior will be when asked about his exam results.

5. The student verbalized the blood pressure findings by telling the patient, "Your blood pressure is 126 over 82." He then asked, "Is that about normal for you?" This form of verbalization is acceptable to the FTO.
   a. True
   b. False

   The correct answer is **a**. This form is not only acceptable; it is the most efficient form of student verbalization.

Briefings and Verbal Feedback

KEY POINTS

- Daily briefings tell the student "This is what I expect you to do today."
- Daily briefings preempt student excuses.
- Briefing the partner decreases the number of inadvertent prompts.
- Verbal feedback helps students avoid repetitive mistakes.

This chapter offers a few techniques to improve FTO–student communication. Students perform more effectively when they understand exactly what they are expected to do. FTOs use briefings and verbal feedback to communicate expectations to students. Verbal feedback will decrease repetitive student errors.

Briefings and verbal feedback remind students of their team leadership responsibilities. FTOs also use briefings and verbal feedback to preempt student excuses. These techniques are designed to speed up the learning process. When students learn more quickly, and when students do not make excuses, an FTO's job will be simplified.

Students should be briefed at the beginning of each day. During this briefing, FTOs remind students of their team-leader responsibilities. FTOs should also ask the students if they have any questions about the field internship process. By doing so, FTOs can lay the groundwork to refute any excuses the student might be tempted to offer.

Student Excuses

Students may use a variety of excuses:

- I didn't know what you wanted me to do."
- "None of the other FTOs want me to do it that way."
- "We don't do it that way back home."
- "I did that. You just didn't see me."
- "I said that. You just didn't hear me."
- "I was just going to do that when you interrupted me."
- "I was just going to do that when your partner did it."
- "I was just going to do that when you (the FTO) did it."

Excuses waste everyone's time and do not solve problems. Briefings *do* solve problems.

Each FTO will have a unique method for prompting students. Students must be able to recognize these prompts. Students must understand what they are supposed to do when prompted by the FTO. FTOs brief students at the beginning of the day so they can avoid hearing excuses.

FTOTips ☑️

Make sure the student understands that excuses are a waste of everyone's time, and will not be tolerated by the FTO.

I Didn't Know What You Wanted Me to Do

Consider the FTO's explanation of how she uses physical prompts: "I prefer using physical prompts. If that fails, or is not suitable for a particular situation, I will use a verbal prompt. You must look around periodically during the patient contact. I will try to position myself where the patient cannot see the prompts. I will stay out of the patient's line of sight so that I do not disrupt your interaction with the patient. Here are some of the prompts I will use:

- Two curved fingers means apply nasal cannula (**Figure 7-1**)
- Cupped hand means apply nonrebreather.
- Two fingers 'walking' means it is time to go.
- Hands in a 'T' means time-out, or hold up for a minute.
- Hand extended upright means stop immediately.
- Circling finger means look around.
- Taking my own pulse means take patient's pulse.
- Showing you my stethoscope means do lung sounds now."

The FTO also explains how she uses verbal prompts: "Sometimes I will not be able to use a physical prompt. Let's say that I want you to ask a specific history question. It's unlikely that I could give you a physical prompt for this question. My prompt will be when *I* ask the question. Or, let's say that I need you to stop doing something and you are not looking at me. I will have to say something to you. If possible, I will always try to use a question when I'm giving a verbal prompt. Here are a few of the ways that I might prompt:

- For application of oxygen, I'll ask, 'How many liters for the oxygen?'
- For pulse rate, 'What did you get for the pulse?'
- For lung sounds, 'What lung sounds did you hear?'
- For pertinent negative history questions, 'Sir, are you having (chest pain, etc.)?'
- For protocol selection, 'What do you plan to do next?'
- To keep you from committing a medication error, 'What medication is that?' 'How much are you giving?' Or, if I absolutely have to, I will say 'STOP!'

"I generally give verbal prompts by asking a question. The patient will think that you are in charge and that I am asking you for an opinion, or that I am just asking you to share the results of exam procedures. The patient will be more likely to

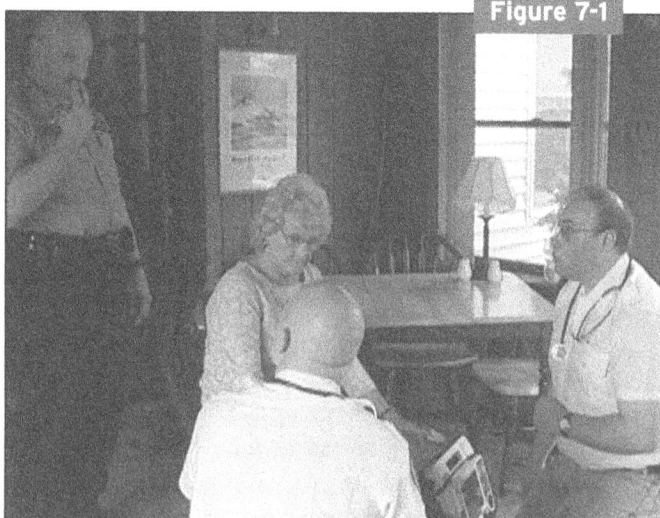

The FTO indicates to the student that he should apply a nasal cannula.

Figure 7-1

communicate freely with you as long as he thinks you are the person responsible for making the decisions."

The FTO has explained how she will prompt the student. This means she should not have to listen to the student say, "I didn't know you wanted me to do it that way." The FTO can continue the briefing by addressing other potential student excuses.

None of the Other FTOs Want Me to Do It That Way

To counter this excuse, the FTO should say, "I'm telling you now that I do not want to discuss how other FTOs do things. It is not appropriate for me to discuss what other FTOs do. You have a copy of the rules, and I have a copy of the rules. We are going to follow those rules. You may have some questions about the rules found in the manual. If you have any questions, ask them now."

I Did That, You Just Didn't Hear (or See) It

The FTO should say, "It is your responsibility to verbalize. Take the pulse rate and tell me what the results are. Listen to lung sounds and tell me what you heard. Tell me what protocol you intend to follow. Always remember that a large portion of your verbalization can be accomplished by reporting results to the patient. Any skill performance you delegate should be assigned to a particular person. Do not say 'somebody take c-spine.' You will not have to verbalize answers to history questions. Just ask the question. I will nod or give a thumbs-up to indicate that I heard the question, and the patient's answer."

I Was Just Going to Do That When You Prompted Me

The FTO should say, "Remember the limits for elapsed time. I do not want to hear you say that you were just getting ready to do something. I will use the time limits from the manual. Let's say that you found evidence of respiratory distress in the initial assessment. At 30 seconds of elapsed time I will prompt you to apply oxygen. Let's say that you have not verbalized a protocol selection at 3 minutes of elapsed time. I will ask you what protocol you have selected. These prompts will be documented on the critique form for that patient contact."

FTOTips ☑

Remember to track elapsed time closely. It affords the student enough time to perform skills, without allowing so much time that patient care will be delayed.

Briefings

Briefings may change as the student moves from one phase of the field internship to the next. The FTO uses briefings to explain the expectations for each phase of instruction. These briefings are relatively simple and straightforward. For the observation phase, the FTO might include the following comment:

- "You (the student) will be observing today. I will be demonstrating how you are expected to do things when you become the team leader. I'll demonstrate how you should verbalize. Feel free to ask questions whenever I do something that you do not understand. I will also delegate certain skills for you to perform. This will give you the opportunity to begin working as part of our team."

For the instruction phase, the FTO might include the following comment:

- "You (the student) are expected to perform as the team leader now. I will prompt you when there is something you need to get done. These prompts are designed to help you provide good care for your patients and to learn when and how certain skills should be done. It is my responsibility to make sure that care of the patient is timely and appropriate. I will use prompts to make sure things get done at the right time. I will use prompts to make sure skills are performed correctly and safely. Each of these prompts will be documented on a critique form. You can receive as many as three prompts and still get a satisfactory score on any patient contact. Do not panic when I prompt you. Prompts are simply a part of the learning process. You will get many prompts early in the instruction phase. The number of prompts should decrease as you gain more experience."

For the evaluation phase, the FTO might include the following comment:

- "You are in the evaluation phase now. The patient contact will be scored unsatisfactory if I have to give more than one prompt. Your percent success rate may drop at the beginning of this phase. Don't panic. Your success rate will probably increase as you get more experience. Do you have any questions?"

Briefing Your Partner

The FTO's partner should be briefed before the student comes to work on the unit. The FTO needs to make sure that the partner understands this process of instruction and evaluation before the student arrives. The FTO's partner is likely to have some questions about how instruction and evaluation of students will impact patient care. The FTO will be very busy once the student becomes a member of the crew. It will be easier for the FTO to answer the partner's questions before the student arrives.

When briefing a partner, the FTO might include the following comments:

- "We are going to have a student with us tomorrow. This student is in the instruction phase of his field internship. I will not let the student do anything that will harm the patient. I will be giving verbal and physical prompts to the student. Here are some examples of what I mean by prompts." The FTO will then demonstrate some of the prompts to be used.
- "The student has time limits for most of the skills he is expected to perform. These time limits are designed to make sure that patient care is not delayed. I will track the elapsed time closely. When we get to the maximum allowable time I will prompt the student to take the correct actions."
- "The student is going to be the team leader for all patient contacts. Neither of us should take over unless the student loses control of the call. I'm going to ask you not to say or do anything that prompts the student. There will be occasions when you just won't be able to resist the urge to perform a skill. You will begin assessing or treating the patient. Your actions will probably remind the student about something that he should be doing. For example: What do you think will happen if you start to get a nasal cannula out of the oxygen bag? The student will see what you are doing. He will then ask you to apply oxygen to the patient. When you open the oxygen bag, the student is prompted to take action. This is an example of an inadvertent prompt. I will then have to make a decision about whether to count this prompt. In most cases I will include this prompt in the total number of allowable prompts that the student can receive for that patient contact. That inadvertent prompt could cause the student to receive an unsatisfactory score for that patient contact. It will be better if you let me prompt the student when his limit for elapsed time has expired. I really need to see if he is capable of making his own decisions."
- "I will sometimes call on you for help. I might ask you to confirm whether a student did, or did not do, something history questions or exam procedures. I simply cannot track everything that goes on one hundred percent of the time. Occasionally, I will need a second set of eyes and ears."
- "Please let me know if you have questions about any part of this process. Ask me about anything that is not clear to you, or anything that causes you to

worry. I know that this process may take some getting used to. I think you will become more comfortable with this process after you get a chance to see it work. I want to thank you in advance for your patience."

The FTO will know what other issues need to be addressed. The FTO's partner will make specific comments and ask specific questions. These comments and questions will lead the FTO in the appropriate direction.

Giving Verbal Feedback to the Student

If everything in life worked perfectly, the FTO would never have to give verbal feedback. In a perfect world, the student would team-lead the patient contact. The FTO would then write the performance evaluation (critique form) for that patient contact. The student would read the performance evaluation and then the FTO would sit down with the student and review it.

Unfortunately, the world is not perfect. It is certainly not going to be perfect for the FTO. The student is not the FTO's only responsibility. The FTO may not have enough time to complete the critique form if the crew is assigned immediately to another call. Life isn't perfect for the student either. Even if the FTO finishes the critique form, the student may not get a chance to read it because he has to clean and restock equipment. This is where verbal feedback comes into play.

The FTO uses verbal feedback to make sure the student has the opportunity to avoid repeating the mistakes from the previous patient contact. The FTO uses verbal feedback as a stop-gap measure when there hasn't been time to complete the critique form.

The FTO gives verbal feedback to the student after the patient has been delivered to the hospital and before the next patient contact. The FTO wants to make sure that the student does not repeat the mistakes made on the last patient contact. But, couldn't the FTO just wait and write all of the comments and suggestions on the critique form?

The FTO could wait, but verbal feedback can provide an effective quick-fix. The FTO can usually give verbal feedback in less than a minute. The FTO wants to make sure the student knows what he did well. The FTO also wants the student to know what skill performances need to be improved. The FTO wants to pass this information along while the student's memory of the patient contact is still fresh and before the opportunity to give feedback is lost.

The crew may get another call if the FTO waits too long to give feedback. The FTO may lose an opportunity to teach. Certain things must be done before the crew is ready to respond to the next call. The FTO should give the student verbal feedback before either of them gets tied up with other work.

Verbal feedback must be a private discussion between FTO and student. Information about the student's scores/grades should always be kept confidential. It is the FTO's responsibility to respect the student's right to privacy.

Verbal feedback follows a simple format. The FTO might begin by briefly explaining what skill performance was satisfactory. This positive feedback will help temper the student's reaction to the negative feedback that will follow, if any is necessary. The FTO should then explain what skill performance was unsatisfactory. The FTO can then make recommendations for improving the student's performance. The student can use these recommendations to keep from repeating the mistakes that have just been made. The student is afforded the opportunity to ask questions.

FTOTips ☑

Give verbal feedback as soon as possible following completion of a patient contact. The student should use this information to avoid making the same mistakes on the next call, and positive feedback will affirm excellent care techniques.

Verbal Feedback Scenarios

Scenario 1

The patient is a 23-year-old female who complained of shortness of breath. Her rate of breathing was very fast. The student stated that the patient is breathing fast, is in a tripod position, and has retractions. He decided to apply supplemental oxygen using nasal cannula. The FTO prompted the student to use a high-flow nonrebreather device instead.

Further assessment and treatment was accomplished without prompting from the FTO. The patient was delivered to the hospital and transfer of care was completed. The FTO then brings the student to an area where they can have a private discussion.

(FTO): "I'd like to give you some feedback."

(Student) "OK. I want to know what I did wrong."

(FTO) "Most of the assessment and treatment for your last patient was performed satisfactorily. I did give you one prompt. During the initial assessment, you said that she was breathing very fast. You also said she was sitting in a tripod position and had retractions. You asked Joe to apply a nasal cannula, and then you began to assess circulation. That is when I prompted you to apply oxygen via a nonrebreather mask. This patient exhibited signs that are consistent with someone who is working very hard to breathe. You should always use a high concentration of oxygen to patients that are working that hard to breathe. Do you have any questions?"

The student replies that he does not have any questions. He says that he will not make the same mistake again. The FTO has given verbal feedback. The student should now be prepared to treat severe respiratory distress even if it occurs on the very next call.

Scenario 2

The patient is an 18-year-old female who has been involved in a motor vehicle crash. Both sides of the vehicle and the roof have experienced significant damage. The vehicle was in the upright position upon EMS arrival. The patient was ambulatory and denied having any pain even though she had a large contusion on her forehead. The student began asking the patient questions related to the mechanism of the crash.

The FTO prompted the student to delegate c-spine control and to initiate an initial assessment. Further evaluation and treatment was accomplished without prompting from the FTO. The patient was delivered to the hospital and transfer of care was completed.

The FTO's partner began restock and cleanup. The student started working on the patient care report. The FTO spent 5 minutes completing the critique form for this patient contact. The FTO then gave the following verbal feedback:

(FTO) "If it's OK, I need to talk about the patient we just brought in. There were several things that concerned me."

(Student) "It's OK. I need to know what I did wrong."

(FTO) "First, you did not verbalize that you noted damage to the patient's vehicle as we approached the scene. Damage to the roof, and to both sides, is a sign of a rollover. That is a sign of significant mechanism! Second, c-spine control is necessary for patients involved in crashes with significant mechanism, especially when there are signs of obvious injury. Third, you cannot delay the initial assessment just because the patient is ambulatory."

The FTO then asks if the student has any questions. The student replies that he had not looked that closely at the vehicle as they approached the last scene. He says that he will not make that mistake again.

Scenario 3

The patient is a 55-year-old male who complained of chest pain and dizziness. During the initial assessment, the patient's rate of breathing was found to be faster than normal. The FTO prompted the student to apply supplemental oxygen. The patient's radial pulses were found to be weak. His skin was pale, moist, and cool to the touch. The FTO prompted the student to lower the patient's head. She also prompted the student to delegate someone to write down a list of medications while the patient was being loaded onto the stretcher. Further evaluation and treatment was accomplished without prompting from the FTO.

The patient was delivered to the hospital. The FTO's partner began working to prepare the vehicle and equipment for the next call. The FTO and the student began to restock equipment and supplies.

The FTO used this time (during restock) to give confidential verbal feedback to the student.

(FTO) "I want to make sure that you understand why I gave three prompts on that call. Some of the patient contact was completed satisfactorily. Unfortunately, I had to prompt you to perform some very important skills: I prompted you to give oxygen because the patient was breathing quickly. I prompted you to lower the patient's head because he was dizzy, and had weak radial pulses. I prompted you to delegate someone to get the medication list so that we would not have to delay transport once the patient was loaded on the stretcher."

The FTO now asks the student if he has any questions about these prompts. The student replies that he understands about the oxygen and the medication list. He does not understand why the FTO wanted him to lower the patient's head. The FTO replies, "Your patient stated that he felt dizzy. He was pale and cool to the touch. He also had weak radial pulses. These signs and symptoms are typical for someone who has a low blood pressure. We lower the patient's head to promote better blood supply to the brain."

The FTO has given the student verbal feedback and answered all related questions. The student should now be able to respond appropriately, even if the very next patient presents with similar signs and symptoms.

Verbal feedback provides important information to the student. The FTO uses this feedback as a temporary solution. The FTO gives this feedback whenever there will be a delay in completing, and discussing, the critique form for a certain patient contact. The student can then use this (verbal feedback) information to avoid repeating mistakes made on previous patient contacts.

Check Your Knowledge

1. The FTO should brief the student at the beginning of each day. This briefing is a reminder of exactly what the FTO wants the student to do. What is the goal of this briefing?
   a. To help the student improve his performance
   b. To remind the student not to make excuses
   c. To answer any questions the student might have
   d. All of the above

   The correct answer is **d**. Daily briefings are designed to improve student performance. They also remind the student not to waste time making excuses. The briefing also gives the student a chance to ask questions.

2. FTOs should brief their partners before students come to work on the unit.
   a. True
   b. False

   The correct answer is **a**. The FTOs should brief their partners before students arrive. This gives the partner time to think about the process and to ask questions.

3. The FTO gives verbal feedback _____ the patient has been delivered to the hospital and _____ the next patient contact.
   a. before, after
   b. before, during
   c. after, during
   d. after, before

   The correct answer is **d**. The FTO should give verbal feedback shortly after the patient has been delivered to the hospital. Feedback should be completed before the next patient contact. The student can then use this information to avoid repeating errors made on the last call.

4. Verbal feedback is designed to eliminate repeated mistakes by the student. It is used as a temporary solution whenever there is a delay in completing and discussing the performance evaluation for that patient contact.
   a. True
   b. False

   The correct answer is **a**. Verbal feedback fills the gap that occurs when the FTO may not be able to complete the performance evaluation. The FTO gives a short synopsis of the preceding call, explaining any mistakes the student made. The student uses this information to avoid repeating these errors on the next patient contact.

Confirming Physical Examination Findings

- Students are required to demonstrate proficiency in physical examination skills.
- Examination findings are only considered accurate if they are confirmed by the FTO.
- FTOs cannot confirm student exam findings unless they are positioned properly.

This chapter offers techniques for confirmation of physical examination findings, such as pulse, respiratory rate, blood pressure, and lung sounds. It is important for the FTO to be in the right place, at the right time, in order to confirm a student's examination findings.

Scenarios

The Student Performs an Accurate Physical Examination

The student is required to demonstrate proficiency as a team leader. Multitasking is a key component of the student's ability to team-lead. The student demonstrates the ability to multitask by performing exam procedures while communicating with the patient and other providers. The student's ability to multitask is demonstrated by performing exam procedures correctly. How does the FTO determine whether the student's findings (pulse rate, blood pressure, etc.) are accurate?

The FTO starts by making sure she is in the right place, at the right time. Positioning is important, and techniques for positioning are presented later in this chapter. But is it really necessary for the FTO to confirm the student's findings? Any student can take a pulse, right?

Actually, the student must *prove* that he is able measure the patient's pulse rate. The student must prove that he can take an accurate blood pressure. The student must also show that he can identify "wheezes" when he is checking the patient's lung sounds. An FTO who is positioned correctly will be able to determine whether the student is having problems performing any of the various physical exam skills. If a student is having problems, a properly positioned FTO will be able to help the student problem solve. And, it is very likely that there will be problems!

The student will make mistakes from time to time. He may get a pulse rate that is not accurate. His findings for the respiratory rate may be wrong. He may identify lung sounds incorrectly. The FTO will know the student's findings are wrong when she compares her own exam findings with those of the student.

The Student's Examination Findings Are Not Correct

The FTO knows what the *correct* findings are because she completed her own exam. The student announces that the patient's pulse is 56, but the FTO has counted a pulse rate of 72. The FTO can now ask the student to recheck the pulse rate. The FTO wants the student to correct his mistakes. In order to accomplish this goal, the FTO first needs to find out what caused the student's error. Some common causes of student mistakes can be found on the following pages.

This all sounds like a lot of work for the FTO. Is all of this work necessary? Will the FTO be required to confirm *all* of the student's exam findings?

No, the FTO is not required to confirm each and every student examination finding. FTOs will, however, need to confirm a significant portion of student findings. An FTO needs to know whether the student is capable of consistently performing an accurate physical exam. The student has to demonstrate that he can take an accurate pulse. He must demonstrate the ability to take an accurate blood pressure. He has to demonstrate the ability to accurately interpret lung sounds. The only way an FTO can be sure a student's findings are consistently accurate is by confirming a significant portion of those examination results.

The FTO may elect to spot check the student's findings. Spot checks can reduce the amount of time an FTO spends monitoring student performance. Once the student has demonstrated proficiency in certain skills, the FTO can use spot check confirmations to make sure the student stays on target.

Techniques for Confirming Physical Exam Findings

Confirming the Pulse Rate

Timing is important. The FTO should count the pulse rate at the same time the student is counting. It is not unusual for a pulse rate to vary over the course of a patient contact. The FTO will only be able to verify the student's findings if both the FTO and the student are checking at the same time.

The FTO should let the student select where to check the pulse. Then, the FTO can count the pulse rate on the opposite arm or on a leg. This method works well for pulse points such as radial, brachial, or pedal pulse points (**Figure 8-1**).

Occasionally, the student's findings will be incorrect. The student may have trouble finding the pulse point. The student may not know exactly how much

FTOTips ☑

The FTO should confirm exam findings at the same time the student performs his exam. For example, findings such as pulse rates, respiratory rates, and lung sounds may change radically over a relatively short period of time, making confirmation findings useless.

Confirming a radial pulse.

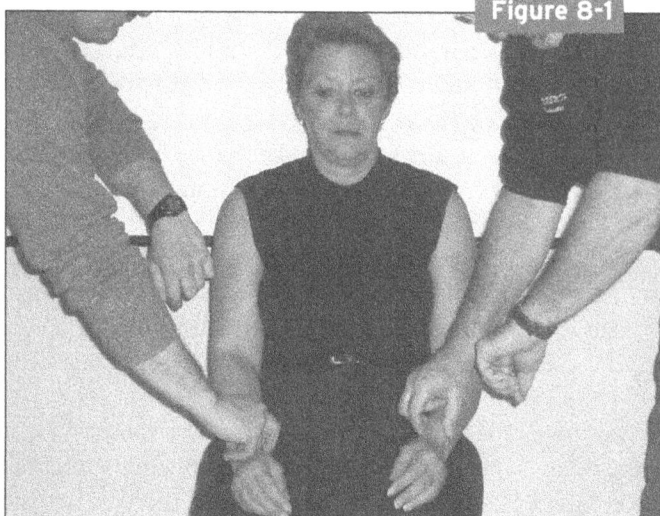

Figure 8-1

pressure to use when palpating for the pulse. The student may make a simple math error in multiplication. The chapter on prompting provided examples of how FTOs can use each of these situations as an opportunity to teach. The FTO can explain how the pulse feels ("It's fast; it's strong; it's regular."). The FTO can show the student where she is palpating. The FTO can check the student's multiplication.

The FTO's best opportunities to teach occur when both the FTO and the student are checking the pulse simultaneously. The same principle can be applied to most techniques that FTOs use to confirm physical exam findings.

Confirming the Respiratory Rate

Once again, timing is important. The FTO should count the respiratory rate while the student is counting. It is not unusual for the respiratory rate to vary throughout the course of a patient contact. The FTO will only be able to verify the student's findings if FTO and student are counting at the same time.

Many students are taught to count the respiratory rate as soon as they are finished counting the pulse rate. The FTO should use the same technique the student is using. This allows an accurate comparison to be made between the FTO's findings and the student's findings.

What should the FTO do on those occasions when the student's findings are not accurate? The FTO should ask the student how he got that rate. The FTO needs to determine if the student is having trouble visualizing the patient respirations or if the student has made some other error. Once the FTO understands the problem, an explanation of how to correct it can be provided.

For example, what if the student is accurately identifying each of the patient's ventilations, but was unable to give the rate correctly? The student is probably making a simple error in multiplication. Maybe the student is having trouble visualizing the patient's respirations. The FTO can help the student correct a problem the cause of the mistake has been determined.

Confirming the Blood Pressure

Timing is also important in this situation. Blood pressure often varies throughout the course of a patient contact. For this reason, the FTO should confirm findings at the same time the student performs the skill. Several options are available for verifying the student's blood pressure results:

- The FTO can place her stethoscope adjacent to the student's stethoscope. The FTO allows the student to select the location where he will listen. The FTO then places her scope next to the student's. This method preempts the excuse "you took my spot." The FTO may find it effective to use a placement that is medial, or distal, to the student's scope. This is the most accurate of the three confirmation techniques provided in this chapter (**Figure 8-2**).

  The FTO may elect to palpate a systolic pressure at the same time the student auscultates for systolic and diastolic pressures (**Figure 8-3**). This technique is only used when the FTO cannot auscultate without disrupting the flow of the patient contact or when the FTO is simultaneously performing another skill. The FTO should remember that a palpated systolic pressure is likely to be several points lower than the student's auscultated systolic pressure.

- The FTO may elect to have the student take the blood pressure and leave the cuff in place. The FTO can then immediately retake the blood pressure. When using this method, the FTO's pressure readings may be slightly higher than the student's. This technique is useful in situations where the FTO simply does not have enough room to utilize one of the other methods.

Note that each of these techniques has limitations. Some might suggest that the

Confirming blood pressure by placing the scope distal to the student's scope.

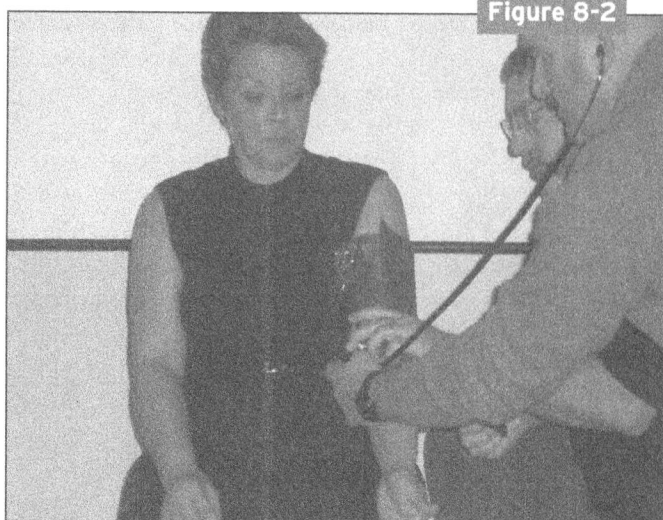

Figure 8-2

Confirming blood pressure by palpating a systolic pressure while the student auscultates.

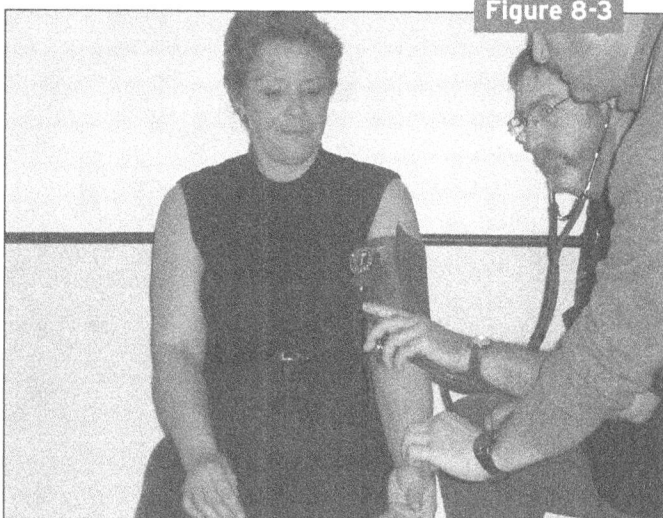

Figure 8-3

use of a teaching stethoscope would yield more accurate results, but our experience has been that a teaching stethoscope is an unwieldy and cumbersome tool, especially in the prehospital environment.

The authors have successfully used the techniques just presented, in both the emergency department and field environments, for more than 10 years. Periodically, FTOs (and clinical instructors) working in the emergency department can demonstrate the validity of their findings (to the students) by following up the FTO's blood pressure findings with findings from a wall-mounted electronic unit. One or two confirmations of this nature normally provide sufficient validation and alleviate any student concerns.

Confirming Lung Sounds

Timing is also important for confirming lung sounds. It is not unusual for lung sounds to change throughout the course of a patient contact. Certain lung sounds may temporarily clear when the patient coughs. Lung sounds may change as the patient's condition worsens. Lung sounds may change as the patient's condition improves. It is important that the student and FTO to listen at the same time.

Lung sounds are evaluated at six points on the patient's posterior thorax. The student positions the diaphragm on the patient's skin. The student begins the lung sound assessment by coaching the patient. For example, the student might say, "I'm going to listen to your lungs. When I say 'breathe,' I want you to take a full breath in and out with your mouth open." The student should not, in most circumstances, ask the patient to take more than six breaths. The student needs to learn how to evaluate lung sounds quickly and without making the patient hyperventilate.

The student begins the assessment by listening at the bases of the lungs. FTOs know that fine basilar rales often clear when the patient takes two or three deep breaths. The student is not likely to hear these rales if he listens first at the apices and then works his way down to the bases.

The FTO has a couple of options for confirming lung sounds. Both methods work well. The first option is for the FTO to place a scope adjacent to the student's (**Figure 8-4**). The FTO should let the student position his scope first. This eliminates the excuse, "You took the best spot and I couldn't hear."

The FTO can also listen at a position that is directly opposite from the student's position. The FTO and student then switch sides as each subsequent breath is taken (**Figure 8-5**).

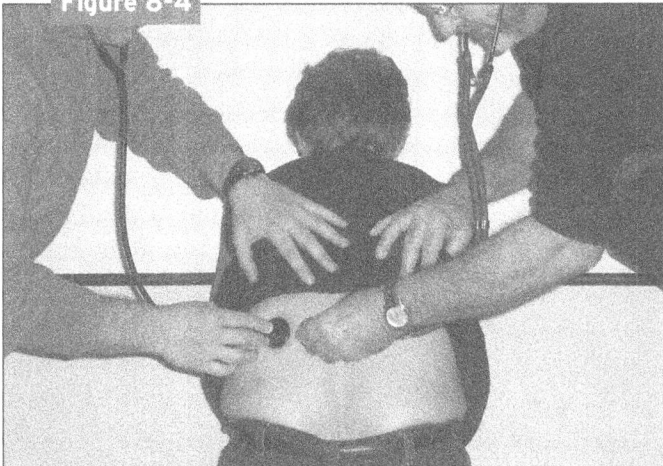

Figure 8-4

Confirming breath sounds by placing the scope adjacent to the student's.

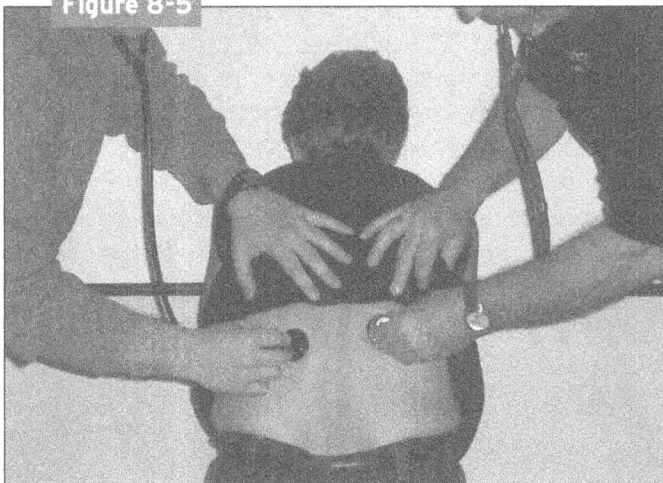

Figure 8-5

Confirming breath sounds by placing the scope opposite the student's.

A Word About Teaching Stethoscopes

Teaching stethoscopes (stethoscopes that have two sets of binaurals so that the student and instructor may auscultate simultaneously) have been used for many years in the clinical setting. The FTO may find these devices counterproductive for a number of reasons. First, the sound does not tend to be of the highest quality. Second, use of a teaching stethoscope does not allow the FTO to easily change position because the FTO is tethered to the student. Third, and perhaps most important, use of the teaching stethoscope leaves no doubt in the mind of the patient, bystanders, and all other providers that the student is, in fact, a student. This may severely undermine the student's ability to grow as a team leader.

Confirming Other Examination Procedures

Pulse rate, respiratory rate, blood pressure, and lung sounds are the most frequently performed exam procedures; however, the FTO will have to confirm additional physical exam procedures.

The FTO confirms some findings by simply communicating with the student. Ideally, the student will verbalize the results of the examination without being prompted by the FTO. The FTO needs to know two things. First, can the student verbalize the results of a certain examination procedure? Second, were the student's findings correct? The FTO is able to confirm these examination findings by asking questions such as:

- What is the pulse oximetry reading?
- What is the cardiac rhythm?
- What do you see on the 12 lead?
- What is the blood sugar reading?

Performance of certain other skills will require the FTO to take a slightly different approach. The FTO confirms other history (and exam) findings by simply monitoring the interaction between student and patient. The FTO will not have to physically confirm these findings. Medical history questions are not physical exam procedures, but are included here for obvious reasons. The following are a few examples of this monitoring technique:

- The student asks a history question, and the FTO listens to the patient's response.
- The student palpates for painful response, and the FTO watches the patient reaction.
- The student checks capillary refill, and the FTO watches the refill time.

The FTO confirms some findings by watching the student interact with the patient. The FTO confirms some findings by listening to the student interact with the patient. The FTO may elect to confirm certain findings by repeating the exam procedure:

- The student reports crepitus, and the FTO palpates to confirm.
- The student reports the presence of subcutaneous emphysema, and the FTO palpates.
- The student reports that the abdomen is rigid, and the FTO palpates.

What do all of these confirmation techniques have in common?

- The FTO has to be positioned correctly in order to confirm student findings.
- The FTO has to be in position at the right time in order to confirm student findings.
- The FTO's confirmation should not undermine the student's ability to team-lead the contact.

The FTO should establish a position that does not disrupt the flow of the patient contact. However, if the FTO is not in the right place, at the right time, the FTO will not be able to confirm the student's skill performance (**Figure 8-6**). In many ways, the FTO is like a referee in a boxing match.

> ## FTOTips ☑
>
> The FTO will be able to confirm many of the student's findings by simply monitoring the interactions between the student and the patient.

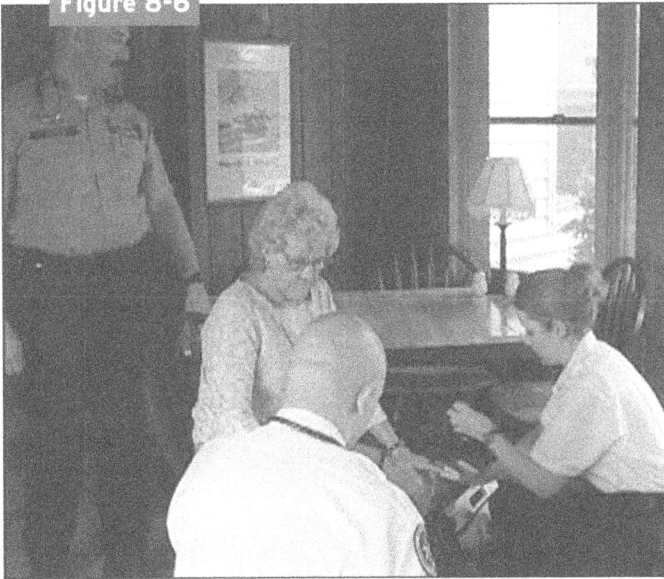

Figure 8-6

The FTO positions himself during the patient contact.

Like a Referee in a Boxing Match

What does a boxing referee do? He motions the boxers to begin fighting when the first bell rings. He makes sure the boxers stop fighting when the next bell rings. He makes sure the boxers play by the rules. He changes position constantly. The referee wants to be in the right place at the right time.

The referee needs to be in a position where he can take corrective action. He moves between the boxers when it is necessary to separate them. He then withdraws quickly so that he does not interrupt the flow of the fight. He also positions himself where he is not likely to get hit.

The referee is not supposed to be the center of attention. Referees and FTOs have similar responsibilities. A boxing match will go as smoothly as possible if the referee does a good job. A patient contact will go as smoothly as possible if the FTO does a good job:

- **The FTO tracks elapsed time, making sure the student doesn't go past the established time limits.** Like a referee, the FTO steps in to prompt if the student is taking too much time.
- **Like a referee, the FTO makes sure the student follows the rules.** The FTO makes sure the student verbalizes; that the student assesses the patient appropriately; and that the student's treatment of the patient is safe, timely, appropriate, and within the local standard of care.
- **The FTO watches the student closely.** Like a referee, the FTO wants to be in position to step in, if necessary. The FTO must be in position to intervene if the student attempts to do something that might harm the patient.
- **The FTO moves quietly and with subtle movements.** Like a referee, the FTO doesn't want to interrupt the flow of the "fight," or patient contact in this case.
- **Sometimes the FTO will have to prompt the student.** The FTO will give the prompt and then, like a referee, quickly withdraw.
- **Like a referee, the FTO changes position constantly.** The FTO has to be in position to confirm a student's assessment findings. The FTO moves so that she can see the patient. The FTO moves so that she can see monitoring equipment such as a pulse oximeter or cardiac monitor. The FTO moves out of the patient's line of sight so that she can give a physical prompt to the student. She quickly moves to stop the student if he is doing something that might harm the patient.

FTO Tips ☑

Like a referee in a boxing match, the FTO will always want to be in the right place at the right time.

- **Like a referee, the FTO stays in position to make sure that neither patient, nor student, is harmed (hit by a "low blow").**
- **The FTO protects herself from getting hit by one of the boxers.** Anything that goes wrong during the patient contact will end up being the FTO's fault. Like a referee, the FTO will take a "hit" whenever something goes wrong.
- **Like a referee, the FTO isn't supposed to be the center of attention.** The patient is the center of attention. The student is the team leader. The patient's attention should be centered on the student. The student's opportunity to learn from a patient contact will be compromised if the FTO becomes the center of attention.

The FTO is the referee for every patient contact. Teaching and evaluating students is hard work for the referee. FTOs invest a lot of time and effort helping students learn. An FTO can use certain techniques to simplify this process. FTOs will be able to work more efficiently if they are in the right place, at the right time.

Positioning for the FTO

Sometimes the FTO will feel caught between a rock and a hard place. The FTO wants to be able to prompt the student without attracting the patient's attention. The FTO also wants to be in position to confirm a student's exam findings. The FTO wants to make sure the patient contact proceeds smoothly.

Positioning is not difficult when the patient contact occurs outdoors. Plenty of room to operate is usually available at the scene of a motor vehicle crash or at a construction site accident. The FTO will usually have little difficulty finding a good position when the patient contact occurs outside.

For example, say the patient has suffered a cardiac arrest on a golf course. In such a situation, there is plenty of room for all the providers to work. The FTO can adjust position by simply circling around the patient to be in the right place, at the right time. The FTO confirms exam findings, watches the monitoring equipment, and guides the student through skill performances such as CPR, defibrillation, and medication administration.

It is sometimes more difficult to find a good position when the patient is in a building. Every FTO has treated a number of patients in bathrooms and in hallways. Changing positions in these kinds of situations can be challenging.

The FTO can make adjustments in a couple of ways. The FTO may first make allowances with regard to confirming exam findings, accepting the student's findings that there is no carotid pulse when the patient is exhibiting no signs of life. The FTO might defer a confirmation pulse check for a few seconds.

Other adjustments are possible. The FTO could prompt the student to move the patient to a more spacious area. The FTO's effectiveness will be directly related to the FTO's ability to monitor both the student and the patient. This effectiveness will be challenged again as soon as the patient is moved to the ambulance.

The FTO's ability to move around inside an ambulance can be compromised by several factors once the patient has been moved to the ambulance. The FTO will have more room to maneuver in a box-style ambulance. Van-style ambulances tend to have less space available. FTOs should be assigned to box-body ambulances whenever possible. The total number of providers in the patient compartment will also have an impact on the FTO's maneuverability.

FTOs evaluate a student's ability to delegate and multitask. Ideally, the FTO wants to watch the student work with a partner. But, the FTO still needs to be in position to confirm important exam findings and to be in position to intervene whenever the student needs help. This is sometimes difficult in the back of an ambulance.

Two or three seat positions are usually available in the patient compartment. The bench seat is usually adjacent to the patient's left side. This seat usually accommodates two persons and a small amount of equipment. The jump seat (CPR seat) usually has room for one person and is located at the patient's right side. The captain seat is located somewhere between the patient's head and the front compartment of the vehicle and has room for one person.

The FTO should carefully choose her seat location. The FTO will not be able to easily change position when there are more than two providers in the back of the unit. It may be possible for the FTO to change position, but it is frequently a difficult chore.

The FTO should use the captain seat as a last option. The FTO will not be able to see the patient from this position or be able to confirm pulses, blood pressures, or lung sounds. The FTO must be in position to intervene whenever the student needs help.

Because this seat is behind the patient, respiratory arrest might not be witnessed by the FTO. Changes on monitoring equipment such cardiac monitor or pulse oximetry may go unnoticed. The FTO will be unable to confirm vital signs taken by the student. These are just a few examples of why the captain seat is a poor seat for the FTO.

The FTO may elect to sit in the jump seat when acting as the student's partner. Patient care can be provided from this position. Confirmation of exam findings can often be performed from this position. From this position, an FTO can give prompts to the student. Additionally, the FTO will have some freedom of movement from this position, giving the FTO the option to participate in patient care whenever needed.

The FTO should use the bench seat whenever possible, sitting between the student and the rear door of the ambulance. The patient is easily seen from this position. The FTO will be able confirm most exam findings from this position and help the student perform physical skills. The FTO can often assist with patient care from this position. On most occasions, this is the best position for the FTO.

Of course, there are exceptions to any rule. The FTO will have trouble confirming lung sounds from this position and may have to accept the student's findings or ask her partner to confirm the student's findings. The FTO may also choose to sit at the forward end of the bench seat, placing the FTO somewhat diagonal behind the patient. The view of the patient is partially obscured, but can be improved by leaning forward in the seat. This position can be effective for confirming findings and intervening, when necessary. The FTO should try each of these positions to find the one that is most comfortable and effective.

"Murphy's Law" often comes into play for EMS crews. FTOs should not tempt fate. The FTO will frequently wish she was in a better position. Poor positioning could result in harm to patient or provider.

FTOTips ☑

While in the ambulance, the captain seat is the least desirable position for an FTO. From this position the FTO has limited access to both patient and student.

Check Your Knowledge

1. The student's findings for pulse or respiratory rates are sometimes wrong because the student
   a. multiplied incorrectly (made a math error).
   b. had trouble locating the pulse point or visualizing the respirations.
   c. Both a and b
   d. None of the above

   The correct answer is **c**. It is not unusual for a student to make a math error. He may count the pulse for 15 seconds and mistakenly multiply by 2. He may not be capable of multiplying 27 times 4 without using a calculator. The student may also have trouble visualizing each ventilatory cycle. The FTO may have to show the student how to visualize when counting the respiratory rate.

2. The FTO needs to know if the student is capable of getting accurate results for physical examination procedures, such as pulse rate, respiratory rate, blood pressure, and lung sounds.
   a. True
   b. False

   The correct answer is **a**. The FTO cannot help the student correct mistakes without knowing exactly what those mistakes are. The FTO needs to know if a student is having trouble finding the correct pulse point. The FTO needs to know if the student has a stethoscope that is not working properly or if the student has trouble doing math without pen and paper. She needs to know if the student just doesn't know what wheezes actually sound like. The FTO cannot help the student fix a problem without knowing what the problem is.

3. Like a referee in a boxing match, the FTO should not be the center of attention. The FTO should make sure the flow of patient contact is interrupted as little as possible.
   a. True
   b. False

   The correct answer is **a**. The student is learning how to be a team leader and must be able to hold the patient's attention. The student will no longer be an effective team leader if the FTO is the center of attention.

4. In the ambulance, the worst position for the FTO is usually the _____ seat.
   a. captain
   b. jump (CPR)
   c. bench
   d. None of the above

   The correct answer is **a**. The FTO must be able to see the patient and be able to confirm exam findings. The FTO must be able to intervene if the student attempts to do something that may harm the patient. The FTO cannot perform these tasks effectively when positioned in the captain seat.

The Critique Form: A Tool for Documentation

KEY POINTS

- Student performance is documented on a critique form.
- Each prompt is documented on a critique form.
- The total number of prompts determines a student's score.
- Students demonstrate proficiency by team-leading patient contacts.
- Effective team leaders move ahead, simultaneously, on three fronts.

Critique forms were designed specifically to measure a student's ability to team-lead patient contacts. Team-leading students are responsible for making decisions and performing skills during a patient contact. The student's ability to team-lead is a good, and perhaps the best, measure of the student's overall proficiency as an EMS provider. A critique form's overall score is designed to reflect how well a student performed as team leader.

Students perform many skills throughout the course of a patient contact. Each skill is a part of the student's overall performance. Within a critique form, these skills have been separated into groups. Each skill group will be referred to as a *competency group*. FTOs document skill performance within the most appropriate competency group. Competency groups are further separated into two categories: critical and noncritical.

Critical Competency Groups

More weight is given to the critical competency groups when evaluating student performance. Historically, within one statewide EMS system, these critical competency groups have proven to be the most reliable predictors of student success in the field internship. The critical competency groups contain key skills related to the student's ability to gather pertinent information, to make good decisions, to implement appropriate treatment, and to display appropriate behavior. For the purposes of this book, and *only* this particular system of instruction and evaluation, the following competency groups will be considered critical indicators of student performance:

- Scene Management and Multitasking
- Initial Assessment and Initial Interventions
- History
- Physical Examination
- Protocols/Standard of Care
- Reassessment
- Change of Therapy
- Professionalism and Affective Behavior

Noncritical Competencies

Some competency groups are *not* considered to be critical indicators of student performance. These competency groups measure a student's performance of psychomotor and communication skills. They are not weighted as heavily as critical competency groups simply because, historically, they have not been reliable predictors of student success.

Psychomotor skills *are* important components of patient care. So, why aren't they considered critical indicators of student performance? FTOs might be able to think back to that rare occasion when they were unable to get an accurate blood pressure. Maybe there were lung sounds they could not positively identify. Maybe there was an occasion when an IV was missed, and the FTO's partner had to pick up the slack. It happens to every provider. It will certainly happen to students!

The student *is* required to demonstrate a certain level of proficiency when performing psychomotor skills. However, the FTO can expect that a student's ability to perform psychomotor skills will improve at a rapid rate as he gains more experience and more confidence. It is likely that an FTO can teach any student how to perform physical skills, given enough time. The noncritical competency groups are:

- Skills
- Verbal Reports
- Written Reports

Critical and noncritical competency groups make up the bulk of the critique form. Other portions of the form are designed to capture demographic data, to provide reminders to the FTO, and to provide a mechanism for delivering an action plan to the student. Each of these components plays an important role in the FTO's instruction.

Instruction to Students

The FTO is the student's role model, representing wisdom and experience. The FTO has "been there, done that, got the T-shirt." Students want very much to get their own T-shirts as quickly as possible and show they can act like experienced providers.

In order to act like experienced providers, the students must first understand how FTOs makes decisions. On many occasions, a student may be wondering: "How did she do that? How did the FTO know to ask that particular question? What did she see that caused her to do *that* thing, at *that* time?"

Patients receive timely and appropriate care because FTOs are doing the right things, at the right times. As experienced providers, FTOs are very efficient when providing care to their patients. An FTO's approach to patient care resembles an army moving into battle: The FTO is moving ahead simultaneously on three fronts.

Moving Ahead on Three Fronts

The FTO gathers the patient's medical history, performs a physical examination of the patient, and provides care to the patient. The FTO understands that this cannot happen one step at a time: "First, I will get a complete history. Then I will perform a complete physical examination. I will begin treating the patient after I have gotten all possible information." No FTO would take that approach.

An FTO always moves ahead on three fronts. Treatment begins at the same time that history and exam procedures are being performed. How can FTOs teach their students to take the same approach?

The FTO will use prompts to help the student move ahead on all three fronts, teaching the students how to think, and act, like an experienced provider. The FTO will use prompts to motivate the student to do the right things, at the right times, guiding the student through each patient contact.

What happens when the patient contact is over? How can the FTO make decisions about whether a student's performance was acceptable? Did the student pass or fail? The FTO begins making this decision by documenting each prompt that was given to a student. The critique form is where the FTO records any prompts that were given to the student. Each prompt represents guidance the FTO provided to the student. The amount of help (number of prompts) a student requires is a reflection of the student's performance.

Critique Forms

The FTO needs a measuring tool. This tool must be capable of measuring the student's ability to move ahead simultaneously on three fronts. The critique form was designed to be such a tool. The FTO simply makes note of how and when the student was prompted and documents each prompt on a critique form.

The FTO will assign scores (grades) based on the number of prompts that were given to a student. Techniques for scoring patient contacts will be addressed in later chapters.

Critique forms also serve other purposes. They provide a structured template for *how* to teach and evaluate students. They are also templates for students. Critique forms give students a list of the skills that they might be expected to perform. They remind students how much time is allowed when performing certain skills. Critiques are an important tool for both FTOs and students. Examples of critique forms will be shown on the following pages. Each form is a one-page, two-sided, document.

Four sample critique forms can be found on the following pages:

- **EMT-B Field Critique (Form A):** Documents prehospital instruction and evaluation of EMT-Basic students.
- **EMT-P Critique (for Laboratory Scenarios) (Form B):** Documents laboratory instruction and evaluation of EMT-Paramedic students.
- **EMT-P Clinical Critique (Form C):** Documents emergency department instruction and evaluation of EMT-Paramedic students.
- **EMT-P Field Critique (Form D):** Documents prehospital instruction and evaluation of EMT-Paramedic students.

Use Form D as a reference while reading this chapter and the chapters on scoring.

FTOTips ☑️

Whether observing the student during a patient contact or grading his performance afterward, remember to use the four question self-test: Was the student's performance safe? Was it timely? Was it appropriate for this patient contact? Was it within local standards of care? This simple guide will help the FTO decide to prompt or to count a prompt as a teaching point.

EMT-B Field Critique

Circle appropriate phrase: Observation   Instruction   Evaluation   *Submit for Review by Coordinator:*   Yes   No

Section 1

Student/Candidate: Station: Date:

FTO: Incident #:   Priority: 1   2   3

Pt. age / sex: CC :

Pt.'s Presentation, HPI, MOI:

Section 2   Score of: 1 = Unsatisfactory   2 = Unsatisfactory (parts satisfactory)   3 = Satisfactory

FTOs: *Circle the word "Prompt" (and the skill that was prompted) to indicate that a prompt was given.*
         Make a checkmark (through the skill) to indicate satisfactory performance of that skill.
FTO Self-test: Were the student's actions: Timely?   Appropriate?   Safe?   Within Protocol?

Scene / Multi-   Assesses scene safety, need for additional personnel, and takes appropriate actions. Document ability to delegate, to multitask, and make decisions, here.

1. 1   2   3   (elapsed scene time:)

Prompt: Safety   # of Patients/Personnel   Task Delegation (specify)   Multitasking   Decisions (where to . . . , when to . . .)

Initial   Completes the initial assessment within thirty (30) seconds. Physically intervenes, within thirty (30) seconds, to address problems found during the initial assessment.

2. 1   2   3   (elapsed assessment time:)   (elapsed intervention time:)

Prompt: c-spine   Airway / Reposition / Adjunct   Breathing / O_2 / BVM   Circulation / Flat / CPR   Disability (AVPU)   Expose

History   Obtains chief complaint, pertinent history of present illness, and pertinent past medical history.

3. 1   2   3   Associated Symptoms: CP   SOB   IDDM   H/A   N/V/D   Recent: Trauma   Cough   Fever

Prompt: CC   HPI / PMH   Initial   (O, P, Q, R, S, T, A, M, P, L, E)   Hospital Preference   Other:

Physical Exam   Completes all pertinent components of physical examination.

4. 1   2   3   Stroke Scale   Blood Sugar   Rapid Trauma Assessment

Prompt: P   BP   RR   Breath Sounds   Pupils   Pulse-Ox   PMS   Edema   Palpate   Other:

Protocols/Standard/Care   Intervenes within the framework of accepted medical standards, protocols, and standing orders. EMT, or student, must begin appropriate treatment regimen within three (3) minutes.

5. 1   2   3   (elapsed time:)

Prompt: Knowledge of Protocols   Differential Diagnosis   Implementation

Prepared by B. Nepon and B. Eberly/Bayhealth Medical Center

Reassess	Reassesses, within five (5) minutes, for change in patient's condition or presentation.

6. 1   2   3   ++   (elapsed time:)

Prompt: CC   Initial   Vital Signs   Breath   Sounds   Pulse Ox   Pupils   PMS

Change of Therapy	Changes course of treatment, within thirty (30) seconds, following change in patient's condition or presentation.

7. 1   2   3   (elapsed time:)

Prompt: Knowledge of Protocols   Differential Diagnosis   Implementation

Professional/Affective	Fulfills responsibilities for professional conduct and affective behavior as outlined in the *Manual for Paramedic Students and FTOs*.

8. 1   2   3   ++

Prompt: Honesty   Courtesy   Confidentiality   Accepts Responsibility   Accepts Constructive Criticism

Skill   Skill   Skill
9. 1   2   3   1   2   3   1   2   3
Skill
1   2   3   Prompt:

Verbal Reports	Gives complete report to appropriate staff member of receiving facility.

10. 1   2   3

Prompt:

Written Report	Provides complete documentation on Delaware patient care report form.

11. 1   2   3

Prompt:

Section 3 Overall Score:	Satisfactory	++	or	Unsatisfactory
(Instruction phase)	Were there... > 3 Prompts?		Have there been... > 3 Repetitive Prompts?	

FTO Comments: _____

_____

_____

Student / Candidate Comments: _____

_____

_____

_____

FTO Signature: _____   Student/Candidate Signature: _____   Date: _____

EMT-P Critique   *for Laboratory Scenarios*

Circle each appropriate category: Pediatric   Geriatric   Trauma   Cardiac   Neuro   Respiratory   Gen. Med.   Psych.   OB

Section 1

Name: Date:

Instructor: Priority: 1   1-M   2   3

Pt. age / sex and Presentation (HPI/MOI):

Section 2   Score of: 1 = Unsatisfactory   2 = Unsatisfactory (parts satisfactory)   3 = Satisfactory

Instructors: *Circle both the word "Prompt," and the skill that was prompted, to indicate a deficiency.*
Draw a line / when using the indicated prompts as a record of successful completion.

Scene / Multi-	Assesses scene safety, need for additional personnel, and takes appropriate actions. Document ability to delegate, multitask, and make decisions here.

1.   1   2   3   ++   (elapsed scene time:)

Prompt: Safety   # of Patients/Personnel   Task Delegation (specify)   Multitasking   Decisions (where to . . . , when to . . .)

Initial	Completes the initial assessment within thirty (30) seconds. Physically intervenes, within thirty (30) seconds, to address problems found during the initial assessment.

2.   1   2   3   ++   (elapsed assessment time:)   (elapsed intervention time:)

Prompt: c-spine   Airway / Reposition / Adjunct   Breathing / O_2 / BVM   Circulation / Flat / CPR   Disability (AVPU)   Expose

Focused History	Obtains chief complaint, pertinent history of present illness, and pertinent past medical history.

3.   1   2   3   ++   Associated Symptoms: CP   SOB   IDDM   H/A   N / V / D   (Recent) Trauma   Cough   Fever

Prompt: CC   PPTC   HPI / PMH   (O, P, Q, R, S, T, A, M, P, L, E)   Hospital Preference   Other:

Physical Exam	Completes all pertinent components of physical examination.

4.   1   2   3   ++   Stroke Scale   Blood Sugar   Rapid Trauma Assessment

Prompt: P   BP   RR   Lung Sounds   Pupils   Pulse Ox $EtCO_2$ PMS   Edema   Palpate   Rhythm   12 Lead

Protocols/Standard/Care	Intervenes within the framework of accepted medical standards, protocols, and standing orders. EMT, or student, must begin appropriate treatment regimen within three (3) minutes.

5.   1   2   3   ++   (elapsed time:)

Prompt: Differential Diagnosis   Knowledge of Protocols   Implementation

Reassess	Reassesses, within five (5) minutes, for change in patient's condition or presentation.								

6. 1   2   3   ++   (elapsed time:)

Prompt: CC   Initial   Vital Signs   Lung Sounds   Blood Sugar   Pulse Ox   Pupils   PMS   Cardiac Rhythm   12 Lead

---

Change of Therapy   Changes course of treatment, within thirty (30) seconds, following change in patient's condition or presentation.

7. 1   2   3   ++   (elapsed time:)

Prompt: Differential Diagnosis   Knowledge of Protocols   Implementation

---

Professional/Affective   Fulfills responsibilities for professional conduct and affective behavior as outlined in the *Manual for Paramedic Students and FTOs*.

8. 1   2   3   ++

Prompt: Honesty   Courtesy   Confidentiality   Accepts Responsibility   Accepts Constructive Criticism

---

Communication   Establishes and maintains effective lines of communication.

9. 1   2   3   ++   **Establishes Communication**   **Maintains Communication**

Prompt: Patient   Family   Witness   EMS Personnel   Other Personnel

---

Skill   Skill   Skill

10. 1   2   3   ++   1   2   3   ++   1   2   3   ++

IV / ET Skill   S1   S2   (elapsed time:)   Prompt:

1   2   3   ++   U1   U2

Verbal Reports   (Radio)   Contacts medical control. Gives concise report and requests orders (PRN)

(Transfer)   Gives complete report to appropriate staff member of receiving facility.

11. 1   2   3   ++

Prompt:

Rhythm Interpretation   Correctly interprets rhythm from cardiac monitor.

12. 1   2   3   ++

Prompt: Without Printed Strip   With Printed Strip   Rate   Type of Rhythm

---

Section 3   Overall Score: Satisfactory   ++   or   Unsatisfactory

(Instruction phase)   Were there... > 3 Prompts?   Have there been... > 3 Repetitive Prompts?

Instructor Comments: _____

_____

_____

_____

Student Comments: _____

_____

_____

_____

Instructor Signature:_____   Student Signature: _____   Date: _____

EMT-P Clinical Critique	Obs.	Rem.	TL	TLE

Circle each appropriate category: Pediatric Geriatric Trauma Cardiac Neuro Respiratory Gen. Med. Psych. OB

Section 1

Name: Department: Date:

Instructor: Priority: 1   1-M   2   3

Pt. age   Pt. sex M / F   CC :

Pt.'s Presentation, HPI, MOI:

Other students who witnessed this assessment:

Section 2   Score of: 1 = Unsatisfactory   2 = Unsatisfactory (parts satisfactory)   3 = Satisfactory

Instructors: *Circle both the word "Prompt" (and the skill that was prompted) to indicate that a prompt was given.*
Checkmarks will to indicate satisfactory skill performance.

Self-test: Student's actions: Safe?   Appropriate?   Timely?   Within Protocol?

Scene / Multi-

Assesses scene safety, need for additional personnel, and takes appropriate actions. Document ability to delegate, multitask, and make decisions here.

1. 1   2   3   ++   (elapsed scene time:)

Prompt: Safety   # of Patients/Personnel   Task Delegation (specify)   Multitasking   Decisions (where to . . . , when to . . .)

Initial

Completes the initial assessment within thirty (30) seconds. Physically intervenes, within thirty (30) seconds, to address, appropriately, problems found during the initial assessment.

2. 1   2   3   ++   (elapsed assessment time:)   (elapsed intervention time:)

Prompt: c-spine   Airway / Reposition / Adjunct   Breathing / O_2 / BVM   Circulation / Flat / CPR   Disability (AVPU)   Expose

History

Obtains chief complaint, pertinent history of present illness, and pertinent past medical history.

3. 1   2   3   ++   Associated Symptoms: CP SOB IDDM H/A N / V / D   (Recent) Trauma Cough Fever

Prompt: CC   HPI / PMH   PPTC   (O, P, Q, R, S, T, A, M, P, L, E)   Hospital Preference   Other:

Physical Exam

Completes all pertinent components of physical examination.

4. 1   2   3   ++   Stroke Scale   Blood Sugar   Rapid Trauma Assessment

Prompt: P BP RR   Lung Sounds   Pupils   Pulse Ox $EtCO_2$ PMS   Edema   Palpate   Rhythm   12 Lead

Protocols/Standard/Care

Intervenes within the framework of accepted medical standards, protocols, and standing orders. Student must begin, or verablize, appropriate treatment regimen within three (3) minutes.

5. 1   2   3   ++   (elapsed time:)

Prompt: Differential Diagnosis   Knowledge of Protocols   Implementation

Revised 12-8-2004 by B. Nepon & B. Eberly

| **Reassess** | | | | Reassesses, within five (5) minutes, for change in patient's condition or presentation. |

6. 1   2   3   ++   (elapsed time:)

Prompt: CC   Initial   Vital Signs   Lung Sounds   Blood Sugar   Pulse Ox   Pupils   PMS   Cardiac Rhythm   12 Lead

---

Change of Therapy   Changes, or verbalize change of, treatment, within thirty (30) seconds, following change in patient's condition or presentation.

7. 1   2   3   ++   (elapsed time:)

Prompt: Differential Diagnosis   Knowledge of Protocols   Implementation

---

Professional/Affective   Fulfills responsibilities for professional conduct and affective behavior as outlined in the *Manual for Paramedic Students and FTOs*.

8. 1   2   3   ++

Prompt: Honesty   Courtesy   Confidentiality   Accepts Responsibility   Accepts Constructive Criticism

---

Communication   Establishes and maintains effective lines of communication.

9. 1   2   3   ++   Establishes Communication   Maintains Communication

Prompt: Patient   Family   Witness   EMS Personnel   Other Personnel

---

   Skill   Skill   Skill
10. 1   2   3   ++   1   2   3   ++   1   2   3   ++

    IV / ET Skill   S1   S2   (elapsed time:)   Prompt:
    1   2   3   ++   U1   U2

   Cardiac Monitor Strip:

10-A. 1   2   3   ++

Rhythm Interpretation:

Prompt:

Section 3   Overall Score: Satisfactory   or   Unsatisfactory
(Instruction phase)   Were there... > 3 Prompts?   Have there been... > 3 Repetitive Prompts?

Instructor Comments: _____

_____

_____

Initial here if contact is "Unsatisfactory" based solely on severity of one prompt: _____   *Documentation is required.*

Student Comments:_____

_____

_____

_____

_____

Instructor Signature:_____   Student Signature: _____   Date: _____

EMT-P Field Critique	Obs.	Rem.	TM	TL	TLE

Circle each appropriate category: Pediatric Geriatric Trauma Cardiac Neuro Respiratory Gen. Med. Psych. OB

Section 1

Name: Station: Date:

Instructor: Run #:   Priority: 1   1-M   2   3

Pt. age / sex: CC :

Pt.'s Presentation, HPI, MOI:

Section 2   Score of: 1 = Unsatisfactory   2 = Unsatisfactory (parts satisfactory)   3 = Satisfactory

FTOs: *Circle both the word "Prompt" (and the skill that was prompted) to indicate that a prompt was given. Checkmark will indicate satisfactory skill performance.*

Self-Test: Student's actions: Timely?   Appropriate?   Safe?   Within Protocol?

Scene / Multi-   Assesses scene safety, need for additional personnel, and takes appropriate actions. Document ability to delegate, multitask, and make decisions here.

1.   1   2   3   ++   (elapsed scene time:)

Prompt: Safety   # of Patients/Personnel   Task Delegation (specify)   Multitasking   Decisions (where to . . . , when to . . .)

Initial   Completes the initial assessment within thirty (30) seconds. Physically intervenes, within thirty (30) seconds, to address problems found during the initial assessment.

2.   1   2   3   ++   (elapsed assessment time:)   (elapsed intervention time:)

Prompt: c-spine   Airway / Reposition / Adjunct   Breathing / O_2 / BVM   Circulation / Flat / CPR   Disability (AVPU)   Expose

---

History   Obtains chief complaint, pertinent history of present illness, and pertinent past medical history.

3.   1   2   3   ++   Associated Symptoms: CP   SOB   IDDM   H/A   N / V / D   Recent: Trauma   Cough   Fever

Prompt: CC   HPI / PMH   Initial   (O, P, Q, R, S, T, A, M, P, L, E)   Hospital Preference   Other:

Physical Exam   Completes all pertinent components of physical examination.

4.   1   2   3   ++   Stroke Scale   Blood Sugar   Rapid Trauma Assessment

Prompt: P   BP   RR   Lung Sounds   Pupils   Pulse Ox $EtCO_2$ PMS   Edema   Palpate   Rhythm   12 Lead

---

Protocols/Standard/Care   Intervenes within the framework of accepted medical standards, protocols, and standing orders. Student must begin appropriate treatment regimen within three (3) minutes.

5.   1   2   3   ++   (elapsed time:)

Prompt: Differential Diagnosis   Knowledge of Protocols   Implementation

Revised 12-18-2005 by B. Nepon and B. Eberly

Reassess   Reassesses, within five (5) minutes, for change in patient's condition or presentation.

6. 1   2   3   ++   (elapsed time:)

Prompt: CC   Initial   Vital Signs   Breath   Sounds   Pulse Ox   Pupils   PMS

Change of Therapy   Changes course of treatment, within thirty (30) seconds, following change in patient's condition
                                 or presentation.

7. 1   2   3   ++   (elapsed time:)

Prompt: Differential Diagnosis   Knowledge of Protocols   Implementation

---

Professional/Affective   Fulfills responsibilities for professional conduct and affective behavior as outlined in the *Manual for
                                 Paramedic Students and FTOs.*

8. 1   2   3   ++

Prompt: Honesty   Courtesy   Confidentiality   Accepts Responsibility   Accepts Constructive Criticism

---

Communication   Establishes and maintains effective lines of communication.

9. 1   2   3   ++   **Establishes Communication**   **Maintains Communication**

Prompt: Patient   Family   Witness   EMS Personnel   Other Personnel

---

   Skill   Skill   Skill
10. 1   2   3   ++   1   2   3   ++   1   2   3   ++
     IV / ET Skill   S1   S2   (elapsed time:)   Prompt:
     1   2   3   ++   U1   U2

   Verbal Reports   (Radio)   Contacts medical control. Gives concise report and requests orders (PRN).
                                 (Transfer)   Gives complete report to appropriate staff member of receiving facility.

11. 1   2   3   ++

Prompt:

   Written Report   Provides complete documentation on Delaware patient care report form.

12. 1   2   3   ++

Prompt:

Section 3   Overall Score: Satisfactory   ++   or   Unsatisfactory
(Instruction phase)   Were there... > 3 Prompts?   Have there been... > 3 Repetitive Prompts?

Instructor Comments: _____

_____

Initial here if contact is "Unsatisfactory" based solely on severity of one prompt: _____   *Documentation is required.*

Student / Candidate Comments: _____

_____

_____

_____

Instructor Signature:_____   Student Signature: _____   Date: _____

Explanation of the Critique Form

The remainder of this chapter contains descriptions of each of a critique form's sections. The focus of the descriptions will be on the Field Critique (Form D), because it contains the most detailed list of skills and competency groups.

None of the critique forms should be considered to be etched in stone. Each form is just one of many possible variations of what a critique form could look like. The critique form can be modified by adding, deleting, or modifying parts of the form.

What if your EMS agency does not use a critique form? Examination of the critique form illustrates how tools such as prompts and (student) verbalization can be documented. The critique form also can serve as a guide, or as a reference, for FTOs.

The tips and techniques in this book will help FTOs streamline their instruction, regardless of what form they use to document student performance. Prompts can be used to motivate students to do the right thing at the right time, with or without the critique. Limits for elapsed time can be incorporated into any system of instruction and evaluation, with or without the critique form. FTOs can still self-test their performance by asking the questions presented in Chapter 3, critique form or no critique form.

The critique forms, however, were designed to be an integral part of an effective method for teaching and evaluating EMS students. Critique forms are also structured to serve as a reference tool for the FTO. Additionally, the forms can be useful as teaching templates.

Critiques provide an easy-to-use method for providing written feedback to students. Critiques forms provide data that can be used to trend performance. When used for these purposes, this type of form makes it easier for the FTO to develop a more efficient method for teaching and evaluating.

What follows is a step-by-step look at each segment of the EMT-P Field Critique (Form D). From this point forward, the reader may find it useful to refer to a Form D. It may help the reader visualize each of the form's parts more easily.

Header for the Field Critique

EMT-P Field Critique

Circle appropriate phrase: Observation   Instruction   Evaluation

The FTO circles the appropriate phase of the field internship:

- **Observation.** Student observes as the FTO demonstrates, and explains, team-leader skills. The student is required to perform skills, and the student's performance is documented on a critique form.
- **Instruction.** Student serves as team leader. Student may receive a small number of prompts (e.g., three) and still get a satisfactory overall performance evaluation (score) for the patient contact. The student's score is documented on a critique.
- **Evaluation.** Student serves as team leader. Student may receive a smaller number of prompts (e.g., one) and still receive a satisfactory score on the critique.

Example:

> ### EMT-P Field Critique
>
> *Circle appropriate phrase:*   Observation   (Instruction)   Evaluation

Circle Each Appropriate Category

On the next line of the field critique, the FTO should circle the appropriate patient category:

> *Circle each appropriate category:*   Pediatric   Geriatric   Trauma   Cardiac   Neuro   Respiratory   Gen. Med.   Psych.   OB

Patient categories provide useful demographic information regarding numbers and types of patients. Frequently, more than one category will apply. A 70-year-old female complaining of chest pain and shortness of breath might be categorized like this:

> *Circle each appropriate category:*   Pediatric   (Geriatric)   Trauma   (Cardiac)   Neuro   (Respiratory)   Gen. Med.   Psych.   OB

This patient's age (70) qualifies her as a geriatric patient. Chest pain qualifies her for a cardiac assessment. Shortness of breath qualifies her for a respiratory assessment.

Section 1 of the Field Critique

The first section of the Field Critique (Form D) is used to record any demographic information that will be useful to the program coordinator or the quality improvement manager.

> | Name: | | Station: | | Date: | | | | |
> |---|---|---|---|---|---|---|---|---|
> | Instructor: | | Run #: | | Priority: | 1 | 1-M | 2 | 3 |
> | Pt. age / sex: | | CC : | | | | | | |
> | Pt.'s Presentation, HPI, MOI: | | | | | | | | |

Section 2 of the Field Critique

The second section of Form D addresses two specific objectives. The first is to give the FTO tips for how to use the form. These tips guide new FTOs through the evaluation and scoring process. The tip found in the first line reminds the FTO how this particular scoring index is used.

Section 2	Score of:	1 = Unsatisfactory	2 = Unsatisfactory (parts satisfactory)	3 = Satisfactory

The FTO is reminded that student performance is scored as follows:
- **1 = unsatisfactory performance** (student performance was totally unacceptable)
- **2 = unsatisfactory performance** (overall student performance was unacceptable, although parts of the performance were acceptable)
- **3 = satisfactory performance** (meets or exceeds minimum standard for acceptable performance)

The next tip is found directly below the tip for scoring. It reminds the FTO how to document prompts that were given to a student.

Circle both the word "Prompt" (and the skill that was prompted) to indicate that a prompt was given.

The following example shows how an FTO might use this tip: The FTO prompted the student to ask the patient if the pain radiated anywhere. The FTO also prompted the student to ask if the patient has ever had this pain before. Within the competency for History, the FTO documents the prompt as follows:

History   Obtains chief complaint, pertinent history of present illness, and pertinent past medical history.

3. 1   2   3   **++**   Associated Symptoms: CP   SOB   IDDM   H/A   N / V / D   Recent: Trauma   Cough   Fever

(Prompt:)   CC   HPI / PMH   Initial   (O, P, Q,(R,)S, T, A, M,(P,)L, E)   Hospital Preference   Other:

The next tip reminds the FTO that a checkmark indicates satisfactory performance:

Checkmark will indicate satisfactory skill performance.

FTOs may elect to use checkmarks to give their students positive feedback on satisfactory skill performance. The following is an example where an FTO elected to check those history questions that *were* asked by the student. Prompts for radiation of pain and previous episodes are still circled.

History   Obtains chief complaint, pertinent history of present illness, and pertinent past medical history.

3. 1   2   3   ++   Associated Symptoms: CP   SOB   IDDM   H/A   N / V / D   Recent: Trauma   Cough   Fever

(Prompt:)   CC   HPI / PMH   Initial   (O, P, Q,(R,)S, T, A, M,(P,)L, E)   Hospital Preference   Other:

The final tip in this section reminds the FTO to use the four-question self-test when it is not clear if the student's performance was satisfactory:

Self-Test: Student's actions: Timely?   Appropriate?   Safe?   Within Protocol?

The Remainder of Section 2 (Competency Groups)

The following is an explanation of each of the competencies found within the Field Critique Form. Techniques for assigning scores to each competency will be addressed in later chapters.

Gray shading in this section is a reminder. It marks a competency as a critical indicator of student performance. Critical competency groups are weighted more heavily when evaluating student performance.

Competency Group 1: Scene Management and Multitasking

This competency group measures the student's ability to manage the scene and make decisions. The student must complete a scene survey, evaluate for scene safety, determine the number of patients, and assess for the need for triage. The student must coordinate resources and demonstrate multitasking by both delegating tasks and performing skills. The student must make decisions that are appropriate for this particular patient contact.

Scene / Multi-   Assesses scene safety, need for additional personnel, and takes appropriate actions. Document ability to delegate, multitask, and make decisions here.

1. 1   2   3   ++   (elapsed scene time:)

Prompt: Safety   # of Patients/Personnel   Task Delegation (specify)   Multitasking   Decisions (where to . . . , when to . . .)

- The FTO documents the length of on-scene time (arrival to departure).
- Scene-safety skills include use of body-substance isolation and assessment of the scene environment for safety issues that need to be addressed.

- **The student is expected to call for additional personnel and equipment as dictated by the numbers and types of patients.**
- **The student is expected to delegate tasks.** Appropriate task delegation speeds the delivery of patient care.
- **The student is expected to demonstrate the ability to multitask** (i.e. "Can you apply the oxygen and set up the IV while I finish vital signs and lung sounds?").

Providers are routinely required to make time-critical decisions when they are involved in a stressful situation. This is the first of several competency groups in which the student demonstrates an ability to make decisions in a time-sensitive environment.

Competency Group 2: Initial Assessment and Initial Interventions

This competency group measures the student's ability to complete an initial assessment and to initiate appropriate treatment. A potential injury to the cervical spine or an airway obstruction will require immediate care. Inadequate ventilations and inadequate circulation also require care that is time critical. Recommended time frames for successful completion of this competency are included in the critique form. Thirty seconds is the maximum time allowed to complete an initial assessment that has no abnormal exam findings.

Students are likely to need more than 30 seconds to complete the assessment when a problem is found (c-spine, A, B, C, or D). More time is needed because the student must begin to fix the problem. For example, say a patient has snoring respirations. The student must quickly begin appropriate airway control. The initial assessment cannot be completed until the airway compromise has been addressed. The student has 30 seconds to begin fixing the problem, once a deficit has been found.

The student begins the initial assessment by introducing himself. The student then elicits a chief complaint and makes physical contact with the patient. The FTO begins tracking elapsed time when the student first makes physical contact with the patient. This contact might occur when controlling the c-spine, when checking for a patent airway, when palpating and visualizing the chest for ventilations, or when locating a pulse. The student should not be allowed to delay physical contact unless the scene is not safe.

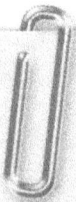

Initial	Completes the initial assessment within thirty (30) seconds. Physically intervenes, within thirty (30) seconds, to address problems found during the initial assessment.
2. 1 2 3 ++	(elapsed assessment time:) (elapsed intervention time:)

Prompt: C-spine   Airway / Reposition / Adjunct   Breathing / O_2 / BVM   Circulation / Flat / CPR   Disability (AVPU)   Expose

Competency Group 3: Gathering the Patient's Medical History

This competency group measures the student's ability to obtain a complete medical history. The student is required to obtain all pertinent history of present illness. This may include the chief complaint, onset, provocation/palliative, quality, radiation, severity, time, associated symptoms, and pertinent negatives. The student is also required to obtain all pertinent past medical history. This may include allergies, medications, previous episodes, last intake/output, and events leading to the problem. The FTO will adjust these requirements in instances where transport time or other factors make it impossible to fully complete this skill. The FTO is the best judge of what history information was pertinent for any particular patient contact.

Consider the following example. The patient is a 24-year-old male complaining of bodywide aches and weakness. The FTO should require the student to ask pertinent negative questions about nausea, vomiting, and diarrhea during the assessment of this patient.

However, a 24-year-old male complaining only of a sprained ankle may not require questions concerning nausea, vomiting, and diarrhea. In most cases, questions about these complaints would not be pertinent.

A patient presenting with altered mental status and who has a history of diabetes would require the student to ask about last oral intake. However, a 50-year-old male with severe, nonreproducible chest pain and no history of diabetes may not require questions about last oral intake.

History	Obtains chief complaint, pertinent history of present illness, and pertinent past medical history.

3. 1   2   3   ++   Associated Symptoms: CP   SOB   IDDM   H/A   N / V / D   Recent: Trauma   Cough   Fever

Prompt: CC   HPI / PMH   Initial   (O, P, Q, R, S, T, A, M, P, L, E)   Hospital Preference   Other:

Competency Group 4: Physical Examination of the Patient

This competency group measures the student's ability to acquire pertinent physical examination findings. The student is required to obtain all physical examination findings that are essential to evaluation and treatment. A number of examination procedures are included in the physical exam competency. Pulse, blood pressure, respiratory rate, and lung sounds are pertinent to the assessment and treatment of virtually every patient. Other examination procedures may be pertinent depending on the patient's presentation. Pertinence of certain procedures will vary in accordance with treatment protocols of the FTO's local EMS system.

For example, consider the following:

- A patient who presents with altered mental status may require a timely blood sugar assessment.
- A patient presents "short of breath and has a history of congestive heart failure." This patient might require evaluation for distal edema.
- A 65-year-old patient with diabetes presents with shortness of breath for the first time ever. This patient may require a 12-lead ECG.
- A 62-year-old patient complaining of a headache and left hemiparesis may require evaluation using a stroke scale.
- An alert and oriented 10-year-old girl who presents with no medical history and a simple fracture of the upper arm does not require a check of her blood sugar.

Physical Exam	Completes all pertinent components of physical examination.

4. 1   2   3   ++   Stroke Scale   Blood Sugar   Rapid Trauma Assessment

Prompt: P   BP   RR   Lung Sounds   Pupils   Pulse Ox   EtCO$_2$ PMS   Edema   Palpate   Rhythm 12 Lead

Components of the physical exam competency group can be modified to meet the EMS agency's particular needs. The previous form excerpt is an example of a physical exam competency group for EMT-Ps. The following is one example of a template for EMT-Bs.

Physical Exam   Completes all pertinent components of physical examination.

4. 1   2   3   Stroke Scale   Blood Sugar   Rapid Trauma Assessment

Prompt: P   BP   RR   Breath Sounds   Pupils   Pulse Ox   PMS   Edema   Palpate   Other:

Competency Group 5: Treatment Protocols or Local Standard of Care

This competency group measures the student's ability to apply the most correct standard of care for each patient contact. The student must provide all necessary interventions within an acceptable time frame. For example, the manual may require students to select an appropriate protocol within the first 3 minutes of the patient contact. The student must verbalize a care plan within 3 minutes. The student is also required to implement treatment within 3 minutes.

Some patient presentations are more complex than others. The student may need more than 3 minutes to determine which protocols are appropriate. In this type of situation, the student is required to verbalize that he is in a "general patient care protocol" before 3 minutes expires. The student should also verbalize a plan for continued patient assessment. This lets the FTO know if the student is on the right track. The FTO can only begin to guide the student in the right direction once the FTO knows that the student is lost.

Prompts for this competency group include the following:
- **Knowledge of Protocol:** Sometimes the student just cannot remember the entire sequence of the protocol. This problem may be resolved by having the student study the protocols.
- **Differential Diagnosis:** Inability to select the correct protocol usually results from the student's inability to diagnose the patient's problem. This may be a warning sign that the student is at risk of failing to complete the educational program.
- **Implementation:** Sometimes the student has trouble implementing patient care. The FTO prompts the student to take action when the student is having trouble getting started.

Protocols/Standard/Care   Intervenes within the framework of accepted medical standards, protocols, and standing orders. Student must begin appropriate treatment regimen within three (3) minutes.

5. 1   2   3   ++   (elapsed time:)

Prompt: Differential Diagnosis   Knowledge of Protocols   Implementation

Competency Group 6: Reassessing the Patient's Condition

This competency group measures the student's ability to reassess the patient in a timely manner. The student is required to periodically reevaluate the patient's complaint and presentation throughout the course of the patient contact. A change in the patient's condition may be a result of treatment interventions. Or, a change in the patient's condition might be caused by continuation of a disease or injury process. The following are a few procedures that are commonly used to reassess the patient's condition:

Five (5) minutes could be the maximum time allowed between assessments. A rapid change in patient condition may require that reassessment be initiated in fewer than 5 minutes. It is the responsibility of the FTO to modify this 5-minute time frame as dictated by patient condition or the scene environment. When a situation arises that requires the FTO to shorten the time frame, the circumstances that required a more rapid reassessment should be documented.

The following is a simplified format for this competency group. This group of skills can be structured to match an agency's level of equipment and operating procedures.

Reassess	Reassesses, within five (5) minutes, for change in patient's condition or presentation.

6. 1   2   3   ++   (elapsed time:)

Prompt:	CC	Initial	Vital Signs	Breath	Sounds	Pulse Ox	Pupils	PMS

The following is a sample EMT-P format:

Reassess	Reassesses, within five (5) minutes, for change in patient's condition or presentation.

6. 1   2   3   ++   (elapsed time:)

Prompt:	CC	Initial	Vital Signs	Lung Sounds	Blood Sugar	Pulse Ox	Pupils	PMS	Cardiac Rhythm	12 Lead

Competency Group 7: Changing Course of Therapy During a Patient Contact

This competency group measures the student's ability to respond appropriately to changes in patient condition. A change in patient condition may require a new course of treatment. The student may be required to quickly alter the course of patient care. This is most likely to occur when there is a rapid change in patient condition. For example:

- Repositioning of the head for a patient whose tongue has become an airway obstruction
- Application of oxygen to a patient who has become short of breath
- Positioning a patient supine following loss of radial pulses
- Removing nitro-paste from the chest of a patient who has become hypotensive

The student might be required to initiate appropriate changes of therapy within 30 seconds. This 30-second time frame begins as soon as the student detects a change in patient condition.

It is not unusual for students to display a poor sense of awareness relative to their environment. Students tend to focus intently on the performance of certain skills (spinal immobilization, wound care, venous access, intubation, etc.). Students' awareness of the scene decreases while they are focusing intently on these skills. They fail to see or hear signs and symptoms related to changes in the patient's presentation. This is one example of when the FTO would be required to prompt.

Change of Therapy	Changes course of treatment, within thirty (30) seconds, following change in patient's condition or presentation.
7. 1 2 3 ++	(elapsed time:)
Prompt: Differential Diagnosis	Knowledge of Protocols Implementation

This competency group is virtually identical to the competency for protocols and standard of care. The FTO still wants to know why the student needed to be prompted:

- **Knowledge of Protocol:** Sometimes the student just cannot remember the entire sequence of the protocol. This problem may be resolved by having the student study the protocols.
- **Differential Diagnosis:** Inability to select the correct protocol usually results from the student's inability to diagnose the patient's problem. This may be a warning sign that the student is at risk of failing the educational program.
- **Implementation:** Sometimes the student needs a prompt so that patient care is initiated in a timely manner.

Competency Group 8: Professionalism and Affective Behavior

This competency group measures the student's ability to act in a professional manner. The student must fulfill the EMS agency's predetermined requirements for affective behavior. The rules for affective behavior will be established by the appropriate local EMS agency. These rules (manual) should be given to the student before the FTO begins to evaluate the student's performance.

Professional/Affective	Fulfills responsibilities for professional conduct and affective behavior as outlined in the *Manual for Paramedic Students and FTOs*.
8. 1 2 3 ++	
Prompt: Honesty Courtesy Confidentiality Accepts Responsibility Accepts Constructive Criticism	

FTOs are sometimes reluctant to document issues related to affective behavior. However, behavioral problems must be addressed in a timely fashion. Poor affective behavior will have a negative impact on the reputation of an EMS agency.

It is not uncommon for students to demonstrate less-than-acceptable affect without understanding what they have done wrong. FTOs should be prepared to help students improve their customer-relations skills.

An FTO may have to prompt the student for deficiencies in the following areas:

- **Honesty:** The student must demonstrate honesty in all areas related to patient care.

- **Courtesy:** The student must be courteous with patients, family, and other providers.
- **Confidentiality:** The student must keep patient information confidential.
- **Accepts Responsibility:** The student must be accountable for his actions. The FTO must not allow the student to make excuses.
- **Accepts Constructive Criticism:** The student must listen to suggestions the FTO offers. The student does not have to agree with everything the FTO says, but the student is required to listen.

FTOs are responsible for helping their students improve their affective behavior. Each act of inappropriate behavior must be documented by the FTO. Prompts given for poor affective behavior indicate that a student may be at risk of failure.

Competency Group 9: Psychomotor Skill Performance

This competency group measures the student's ability to perform psychomotor skills. The following are examples of psychomotor skills that might be included within this competency:

- Acquisition and interpretation of lung sounds
- Application of a cervical collar
- Immobilization of patient on long backboard
- Application of airway adjuncts
- Application of oxygen therapy (NC, NRB, etc.)
- Interpretation of cardiac rhythm
- Establishment of intravenous access
- Tracheal intubation
- Medication administration (IV, IM, PO, etc.)
- Suctioning to clear the airway

This competency group is not considered to be a critical indicator of the student's ability to perform as a team leader. There is no gray shading for this competency. This does not mean that performance of physical skills is not an important part of patient care. It only means that the student should not be given an overall unsatisfactory score based solely on the student's ability to perform psychomotor skills.

The skills competency group for EMT-Bs differs from the format for EMT-Ps. This variation in format is a result of the need to collect data for invasive skills. The FTO writes in all skills except for IV access and tracheal intubation. This allows the FTO to address performance of a variety of skills without wasting too much space on the critique.

The following is a format for EMT-Bs. A few examples of skill performance have been included.

Skill vital signs	**Skill** lung sounds	**Skill** Long board
9. 1 2 ③	1 2 ③	1 2 ③

Skill wound care		
1 ② 3	**Prompt:**	do not remove first pressure dressing, place
see prompt		second dressing on top of first dressing

Examples have been included here simply to show how skills could be evaluated within this competency group. A description of techniques for scoring skill performance will be addressed in later chapters. The circled 3's indicate satisfactory performance of a skill. The circled 2 for wound care indicates that the skill was not performed satisfactorily.

The following is an example of a format that is used for EMT-P students. Examples have been included to demonstrate use. Intravenous access was one of the skills evaluated. The student selected an appropriate vein. His angle of approach resulted in the needle passing through both the top and bottom of the vein. The skill performance was unsuccessful. There was only one IV attempt. The scores and prompts are shown only for demonstration. Specific scoring situations are discussed in later chapters.

Skill	vital signs		Skill	lung sounds		Skill	rhythm interpretation	
10. 1	2	③	1	2	③	1	2	③

IV / ET Skill   S1   S2   Prompt: angle of approach too steep, come
1   ②   3   ⓤ①   U2   in lower so you don't go through vein

- **S1 indicates that a skill was accomplished successfully on the first attempt.**
- **S2 indicates a successful second attempt.**
- **U1 indicates skill performance was unsuccessful, with only one attempt.**
- **U2 indicates skill performance was unsuccessful, with two attempts.**

This provides data the program coordinator will use to determine percent-success rates for certain skills.

FTOs should remember that it is possible for students to have good technique and still not be successful with the skill. A skill may receive a satisfactory "3" even if the attempt was unsuccessful.

The student is required to perform skills within a reasonable amount of time. Patient care may be delayed if the FTO allows the student to take too much time. Recall that elapsed-times were discussed in the chapter on prompting.

Competency Group 10: Giving a Radio/Phone Report to the Receiving Medical Facility

This competency group measures the student's ability to provide a radio or phone report to the receiving medical facility. This competency group should be removed from the critique form if the EMS agency does not routinely give radio reports to the hospital.

Standard reporting procedures will vary from agency to agency. The FTO simply circles the appropriate score and any writes down any prompts that were given to the student.

There is no gray shading on the form for this competency group. These reports are not considered a critical indicator of a student's team-leadership performance.

Verbal Reports	(Radio)	Contacts medical control. Gives concise report and requests orders (PRN).
	(Transfer)	Gives complete report to appropriate staff member of receiving facility.
11. 1 2 3 ++		

Prompt:

Competency Group 11: Giving Report During Transfer of Patient Care

This competency group measures the student's ability to give report at the receiving facility, during transfer of care. The student's report should be accurate and include all pertinent information.

There is no gray shading on the form for this competency group. This report is not considered a critical indicator of student performance.

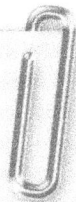

Verbal Reports	(Radio)	Contacts medical control. Gives concise report and requests orders (PRN).
	(Transfer)	Gives complete report to appropriate staff member of receiving facility.

11.   1   2   3   ++

Prompt:

Competency Group 12: Writing a Patient Care Report

This competency group measures the student's ability to document patient-care information on the form designated by their local EMS agency.

There is no gray shading. This report is not considered a critical indicator of student performance.

Written Report   Provides complete documentation on patient care report form.

12.   1   2   3   ++

Prompt:

Section 3 of the Field Critique Form

Overall Score

The FTO reviews the prompts from within each competency group and then selects the appropriate overall score for that patient contact. The FTO circles the appropriate overall score.

Section 3 Overall Score:	Satisfactory	++	or	Unsatisfactory
(Instruction phase)	Were there... > 3 Prompts?		Have there been... > 3 Repetitive Prompts?	

The student receives prompts from the FTO whenever the student needs to move faster. A prompt is also provided whenever the student's assessment and treatment skills are incomplete. Numbers and types of prompts will be used to determine the overall score.

It is possible for a student to receive a satisfactory score even if prompts have been given by the FTO. Section 3 includes a reminder for the FTO to ask the following questions when assigning the correct overall score to this patient contact:

- **Instruction phase:** Were there more than three prompts (> 3 prompts)? The FTO scores the patient-contact satisfactory if three or fewer prompts were given. The FTO scores the patient-contact unsatisfactory if four or more prompts were given.
- **Instruction phase:** Have there been more than three repetitive prompts (> 3 repetitive prompts)? Repetitive prompts occur when the student has been prompted several times for the same thing. When a student receives a fourth prompt for the same skill, it is considered repetitive. Beginning with the fourth prompt, each repetitive prompt will result in an overall unsatisfactory score.
- **Evaluation phase:** Did the FTO give more than one prompt? During this phase, the student might receive an unsatisfactory score if the FTO has given more than one prompt. No reminder is included on the critique form for this situation. Both the student and the FTO will be very familiar with the manual's scoring criteria by the time the student reaches the evaluation phase.

Space for the FTO to Record Additional Comments

Space is also provided for the FTO to record additional comments.

Instructor Comments: _____

_____

_____

Initial here if contact is "Unsatisfactory" based solely on severity of one prompt: _____ *Documentation is required.*

The FTO uses this section to add comments and observations to those already recorded within the individual competency groups on the critique form. The FTO also uses this section to document recommendations for corrective actions. The FTO will advise the student to incorporate these suggestions into an action plan to improve performance.

Space for the Student to Record Comments

Space is also provided for the FTO to record additional comments.

Student / Candidate Comments: _____

_____

_____

_____

The student uses this section to respond to the verbal and written comments made by the FTO. The student also uses this section to respond to the scores entered on the critique form.

The student uses this section to describe any difference of opinion that he has with the FTO. The manual advises students to document any difference of opinion within this section. Note that the student is required to document any difference of opinion before signing the critique.

Signatures of the FTO and the Student

Both the FTO and the student are required to sign the completed critique form. The FTO signs to verify that the scores and comments entered on this critique form are hers. The student's signature verifies that he has read the critique. The student's signature also indicates that he had the opportunity to record his comments on the form. The FTO should enter the date that the critique form was completed.

Instructor Signature: _____   Student Signature: _____   Date: _____

Check Your Knowledge

1. The critique form contains groups of skills that are related, or that are similar. Each of these skill groups is called a *competency group*.
   a. True
   b. False

The correct answer is **a**. A *competency group* is a group of similar, or related, skills.

2. Certain competency groups are considered critical indicators of the student's ability to team-lead a patient contact. Critical competency groups are partially shaded in a gray color.
   a. True
   b. False

The correct answer is **a**. Skills included in a critical competency group contribute heavily to the student's ability to act as a team leader. The top portion of each critical competency group is shaded in gray.

Students rarely fail because they cannot perform psychomotor skills. Students fail because they have difficulty making decisions, they have difficulty making a differential diagnosis, or they demonstrate poor affective behavior.

3. Certain competency groups are related to the performance of psychomotor skills. These skill-groups have no gray shading. They are not considered critical indicators of student performance.
   a. True
   b. False

The correct answer is **a**. Competency groups related to performance of psychomotor skills are not considered critical. They have no gray shading.

4. The student's ability to manage the scene of a patient contact, to delegate tasks, and to multitask is documented in which of the following competency groups?
   a. Initial
   b. Protocol/Standard of Care
   c. Scene/Multi
   d. Skills

The correct answer is **c**. Scene/Multi is a short version for scene management and multitasking. This is a key competency group. This is where the FTO measures the student's ability to make decisions and communicate with team members. The FTO also measures the student's ability to multitask within this competency group.

5. The student's ability to get an accurate accounting of preexisting medical conditions is documented in which of the following competency groups?
   a. Initial
   b. Skills
   c. Physical exam
   d. History

The correct answer is **d**. The History group is where the FTO measures the student's ability to gather a complete medical history.

Scoring the Instruction Phase of the Field Internship

10

KEY POINTS

- The student is learning how to perform in the field environment.
- The FTO's prompts teach the student how to be an effective team leader.
- Each prompt is documented on a critique form.
- The student's overall score is based on number of prompts given by the FTO.
- The student's overall score correlates to the student's performance as team leader.

Chapter 9 reviewed each part of a critique form. This chapter presents examples that show how critique forms are used to evaluate student performance. Critique forms serve as templates that lead the FTO through a simple step-by-step process for scoring.

Scoring in the Instruction Phase

The field internship is where everything starts coming together for both the student and the FTO. The student is beginning to apply didactic knowledge to real-life situations; the FTO is teaching the student how to apply didactic knowledge. The FTO evaluates student performance and assigns a pass-fail score to each patient contact. Critique forms are used create a record of the student's performance. The FTO uses one critique form for each patient contact.

This seems like a lot of work for the FTO. In most instances, it will take less than 5 minutes for an FTO to complete a critique form. Before reviewing some scoring examples, review the following information on prompts and the scoring process.

Why Does the FTO Give a Prompt?

- An FTO's prompts teach the student *how* and *when* to perform a skill.
- An FTO's prompts ensure that patient care is *timely* and *appropriate*.

How Do Prompts Affect a Student's Score?

- Each prompt is documented on a critique form.
- The FTO determines the total number of prompts for the patient contact.
- The FTO assigns an overall score to that patient contact.

How Do FTOs Determine the Overall Score?

Consider a student who is in the instruction phase. He can be prompted as many as three times throughout the course of one patient contact and still receive a satisfactory overall score. Prompts documented in noncritical competency groups are not included in the total number of prompts.

Patient contacts are considered "satisfactory" unless a student receives more than three prompts. FTOs will score each competency group as a satisfactory "3" until the fourth prompt is counted. Four prompts for one patient contact will result in an unsatisfactory overall score. Any score less than "3" indicates unsatisfactory performance.

Consider the following example: A student received one prompt in Initial. Two more prompts were documented in Physical Exam. The fourth prompt for this patient contact was documented in Protocols/Standard of Care. The FTO assigned a score of "2" to the Protocols/Standard of Care competency group because this was the fourth documented prompt on this critique.

The "2" reminds the FTO that the fourth prompt has been documented. It does *not* mean that prompts for protocols are more important than prompts for initial assessment.

The FTO only counts those prompts that are documented within a critical competency group, marked with gray shading.

A student's team-leader performance is scored as either satisfactory or unsatisfactory. The FTO decides whether the student's performance was acceptable. The FTO does not really care if the student can walk on water; the FTO only needs to know if the student can perform acceptably.

Students receive unsatisfactory overall scores when they require too much help from the FTO. The fourth prompt represents too much help from the FTO and results in an unsatisfactory score (2 or 1) in that competency group *and* results in an unsatisfactory overall score.

Review of Scoring Principles

- A student has received more than three prompts. The competency where the fourth prompt is documented receives an unsatisfactory score.
- Unsatisfactory 2 means that some, but not enough, of the skills in that competency were performed satisfactorily.
- Unsatisfactory 1 means that the student's performance was totally unacceptable.
- Prompts documented in noncritical competencies are not included when determining an overall score.

Exception to the Rule (3 or Fewer Prompts = Satisfactory Overall Score)

The FTO always has the option to assign an unsatisfactory overall score, even if there is only one prompt. For example, say the patient's airway was obstructed. The student did not attempt to clear the airway even when prompted by the FTO. This FTO may elect to assign an unsatisfactory score (1 or 2) in the Initial competency based on the gravity of the student's error. Because this is a critical competency, the overall score would also be unsatisfactory.

The FTO is the best judge of the student's performance. The FTO was present when the patient contact occurred. If the FTO's estimation is that one student mistake was sufficient cause for an unsatisfactory overall score, then so be it.

Scoring Examples

The remainder of the chapter contains examples of how to score student performance. At least one example is provided for each competency. At the end of the chapter, two examples of completed critique forms are provided. These sample forms demonstrate how a student's team leadership can be documented on the critique.

Scoring Scene Management and Multitasking

The patient is a 32-year-old male. He presented with a chief complaint of "I can't breathe." The FTO prompted the student to put gloves on before he assessed the patient. The FTO also prompted the student to move the patient out of the cold and rain and into the ambulance.

Scene / Multi-   Assesses scene safety, need for additional personnel, and takes appropriate actions. Document ability to delegate, multitask, and make decisions here.

1.   1   2   ③   ++   (elapsed scene time: *8 minutes*)

prompt to put gloves on . . . prompt to move patient out of rainy weather (2 minutes)

Prompt: Safety   # of Patients/Personnel   Task Delegation (specify)   Multitasking   Decisions (where to . . . , when to . . .)

This FTO documented her prompts within the most appropriate competency group. She circled the words *prompt* and *safety* and *decisions*. Why did the FTO give these prompts to the student? The prompt for putting gloves on was to protect both the student and the patient from a possible exposure to communicable disease. The prompt to move the patient to the ambulance protects both the patient and the EMS providers from bad weather conditions.

Note how the FTO explained the prompts. She explained the safety prompt by writing that she prompted the student to put gloves on. She explained the prompt for decisions by writing that there was a prompt to move the patient out of rainy weather. This FTO also documented the point in time (2 minutes) at which she prompted the student to move the patient.

Each FTO is a unique individual. FTOs will explain prompts in different ways. Some FTOs will use detailed explanations. Other FTOs will save time by using more concise explanations. Let's look at how another FTO might document these same prompts.

> **FTOTips** ☑
> We all appreciate positive feedback. In addition to circling the items that were prompted, the FTO can place a check mark above (or through) items that were completed satisfactorily. This lets the student know that you were watching his performance, and are acknowledging good performance.

Scene / Multi-   Assesses scene safety, need for additional personnel, and takes appropriate actions. Document ability to delegate, multitask, and make decisions here.

1.   1   2   ③   ++   (elapsed scene time: *8 minutes*)

gloves   *move patient*

Prompt: Safety   # of Patients/Personnel   Task Delegation (specify)   Multitasking   Decisions (where to . . . , when to . . .)

Remember that this is an example for scoring one part of a patient contact. Scene-Multi is just one of many competency groups. The student can receive only three prompts and still get a satisfactory score for the patient contact. In the example shown here, the student has already received two prompts.

Scoring Initial Assessments and Initial Interventions

The patient is a 30-year-old female with right-lower-quadrant abdominal pain. The patient was alert and oriented, but had no radial pulses. The student ruled out trauma and determined that the patient was oriented. The airway was patent. The rate of breathing was fast. A prompt was given to apply oxygen.

The student noted that radial pulses were absent. The FTO prompted the student to lower the patient's head. The FTO scored this competency group as an unsatisfactory 2. She elected to assign an unsatisfactory score within this competency group because the prompted skills were such an important part of the patient's care.

The FTO always has the option of scoring a patient contact as unsatisfactory. This may seem to be at odds with the rules for scoring. Why should the student get an unsatisfactory overall score if he received fewer than three prompts?

The FTO is the best judge of what is happening during any single patient contact. The FTO should always have the option to assign an unsatisfactory score to a contact based on the nature of the prompts provided. In this example, the FTO considered oxygen administration and supine positioning to be critical elements of patient care.

Note how this FTO documented the prompts. Also note how the FTO elected to use checkmarks to indicate which skills the student performed correctly.

Initial — Completes the initial assessment within thirty (30) seconds. Physically intervenes, within thirty (30) seconds, to address problems found during the initial assessment.

2. 1 ② 3 ++ (elapsed assessment time: < 30 seconds) (elapsed intervention time: > 30 seconds [B & C])

Prompt: c-spine   Airway / Reposition / Adjunct   Breathing / O₂ / BVM   Circulation / Flat / CPR   Disability (AVPU)   ~~Expose~~

The FTO writes that the initial assessment was completed in less than 30 seconds. The FTO also indicates that the student received a prompt to apply oxygen and reposition the patient. The FTO also uses the elapsed time segments to indicate that the prompt was not given until 30 seconds after each part (30 seconds for breathing, 30 seconds for circulation) of the assessment was completed (> 30 seconds [B & C]). The FTO documents elapsed time to prove that the student had sufficient time to complete the skill.

FTOs might question why they should spend so much time and effort prompting the student. Prompts ensure that patient care will be performed safely. The prompts also ensure that patient care will not be delayed.

Prompts are also an asset for the student. An FTO's prompts teach the student when and how to perform each skill.

Scoring History

The patient is a 65-year-old female complaining of shortness of breath. The patient also appears to have a fever. Five minutes into the patient contact the FTO prompted the student to ask the patient if she has been coughing recently.

History — Obtains chief complaint, pertinent history of present illness, and pertinent past medical history.

3. 1   2   ③   ++   Associated Symptoms: CP SOB IDDM H/A N / V / D Recent: Trauma Cough Fever
at 5 min. early question for Hx of cough may help with lung sounds, and possible Dx pneumonia

Prompt: CC   HPI / PMH   Initial   (O, P, Q, R, S, T, A, M, P, L, E)   Hospital Preference   Other:

The FTO documented this prompt within the History competency group. The FTO also documented why this question was an important part of the patient's medical history. The patient's history of a cough might help the student make a more effective assessment of lung sounds (between rales and rhonchi) or make a more effective differential diagnosis (between pneumonia and congestive heart failure). The FTO noted that the prompt was given 5 minutes into the patient contact. This reminds the student how much time had passed before the prompt was given.

Note that a number of different styles of documentation were used in these examples. This is intentional. The exact method of documentation that individual FTOs use will be the one they are most comfortable with.

Scoring Physical Examination

The patient is an 80-year-old male. He presented with a complaint of "can't breathe." His breathing was rapid, and he was using accessory muscles. The student completed the initial assessment and interventions. The FTO prompted the student to do lung sounds immediately following the initial assessment because of the breathing difficulty. This prompt was documented as shown below, with the FTO circling *prompt* and *lung sounds*.

Physical Exam	Completes all pertinent components of physical examination.		
1 2 ③ ++	Stroke Scale	Blood Sugar	Rapid Trauma Assessment
	teaching point—check for ankle edema early with possible CHF patients		
Prompt: P BP RR **Lung Sounds** Pupils Pulse Ox EtCO₂ PMS **Edema** Palpate Rhythm 12 Lead			

This FTO has also documented a teaching point about checking for edema. Normally this would be written as a prompt. An FTO might elect to make a prompt a teaching point for a number of reasons. Teaching points are most often related to "nice to know," instead of "need to know," information. In this case, the FTO's reasoning was as follows.

It is certainly possible that the student could select the right course of treatment without checking for edema. The FTO's prompt to check for edema should be listed as a teaching point whenever the student is able to make the correct decisions about patient care without requiring information that results from the teaching point (prompt). Teaching points are not counted as prompts, and there is no penalty to the student.

However, checking for edema will sometimes be a very important part of patient assessment. A quick check for distal edema often provides useful information. Presence or absence of edema can be an important part of the physical exam, especially when deciding whether the patient's primary problem is COPD, CHF, or pneumonia. Whenever the inspection for edema is essential to patient care, the FTO will document a prompt instead of a teaching point.

What should an FTO do if the student in this example obtains lung sounds at the right time but incorrectly identifies them? For instance, say the student identifies rales as "rhonchi." The FTO should correct the student's error and explain that these lung sounds are actually rales. How should the FTO document this prompt?

An FTO can document this prompt in one of two ways. The prompt can simply be entered in the Physical Exam competency group. This is a critical competency. These prompts always count when determining the overall score for that patient contact.

The FTO has another option. The critique form was designed to allow FTOs to use their own discretion when documenting performance of any physical skill.

An FTO may believe that the student does not yet have enough experience to differentiate between rales and rhonchi. In such a situation, the FTO can elect to document a lung-sounds prompt within the Skills competency group. The reader will remember that Skills is not considered a critical competency group. Prompts documented in this competency group do not have to be counted when determining the overall score. How would the FTO handle a situation like this? The documentation might look like this:

Physical Exam   Completes all pertinent components of physical examination.

1   2   ③   ++   Stroke Scale   Blood Sugar   Rapid Trauma Assessment
                           teaching point—see skills competency re: lungs sounds

Prompt: P   BP   RR   Lung Sounds   Pupils   Pulse Ox   EtCO₂   PMS   Edema   Palpate   Rhythm 12 Lead

Skill   pulse ox   **Skill**   oxygen/NRB/15 L/M   **Skill**   lung sounds "rhonchi" = rales
1   ②   3   ++   1   2   ③   ++   1   2   ③   ++

IV / ET Skill   S1   S2   (elapsed time:)   **Prompt:** Rales are usually less coarse and are
1   2   3   ++   U1   U2   generally found at the same level in both
                                                                       lung fields.

This FTO is using two shortcuts within the Skills Competency group. Quotation marks are used to indicate that the student said the lung sounds were rhonchi. An equals sign (=) is used to indicate that the lung sounds were actually rales. The FTO then added a short description of rales that may make it easier for the student to identify it.

Scoring Protocols and Standard of Care

The patient is a 20-year-old male who was involved in a high-speed motor vehicle crash. The patient was ejected from the vehicle and landed in a section of soft soil. The patient was alert and was oriented to person and place. Unfortunately, he did not remember what happened or what time it was. The patient repeatedly indicated that he just wanted to go home and did not want to be treated.

The student stated that he was going to allow the patient to sign a refusal-of-service form. The FTO prompted the student to convince the patient to go to the hospital. The FTO also prompted the student to quickly immobilize the patient and begin transport.

Protocols/Standard/Care   Intervenes within the framework of accepted medical standards, protocols, and standing orders.
                              Student must begin appropriate treatment regimen within three (3) minutes.

5.   1   2   ③   ++   (elapsed time: 3 min.)   patient was not oriented to time or circumstance
                             decreased orientation = head injury (?) remember that scene time is limited
                             to 10 min.

Prompt: Differential Diagnosis   Knowledge of Protocols   Implementation

The FTO prompted the student because there was significant mechanism for injury. These prompts also were given because findings of short-term memory loss and repetitive speech patterns indicate a possible head injury. Patients with suspected head injuries need to be immobilized in order to protect the cervical spine. The FTO documented a teaching point by reminding the student that trauma-scene times should not exceed 10 minutes unless there are extenuating circumstances.

A situation like this one may require a more detailed explanation. An FTO can use the section for additional FTO Comments whenever it is necessary to provide a more detailed explanation.

Instructor Comments: I documented a teaching point instead of a prompt for knowledge of trauma protocols. We needed to move quickly so that we could immobilize the patient and get off scene in less than ten minutes. For these reasons I did not give you the opportunity to make these decisions, but made the decisions myself. Consider this a teaching point about protocol knowledge (scene time).   "B"

Notice that this FTO has chosen to personalize her comments with an initial.

Scoring Reassessment of Patient Condition

The patient is a 52-year-old male who was found with an altered mental status. His response to verbal stimulus was slow, but appropriate. Oxygen was administered. His blood sugar was measured at 57 mg/dl. Oral glucose was administered. The patient became alert and oriented over the next 5 minutes. The FTO then prompted the student to recheck the blood sugar.

Reassess   Reassesses, within five (5) minutes, for change in patient's condition or presentation.

6. 1   2   ③   ++   (elapsed time: at 5 min.)
(Prompt:)   CC   Initial   Vital Signs   Breath   Sounds   Pulse Ox   (Glucose)   Pupils   PMS

Notice that the FTO elected to make checkmarks to show which skills the student performed during reassessment of the patient.

Scoring Change of Therapy

The patient is a 26-year-old female who complained of sudden, intense lower abdominal pain. The patient was alert and oriented at the beginning of the contact. Her skin was pale, and she had rapid radial pulses that were normal in strength. The patient was placed on the stretcher and was given oxygen at 4 L/min via nasal cannula.

Five minutes into the patient contact the patient became somnolent and the student reported that radial pulses were absent. The FTO confirmed the absence of radial pulses. Thirty seconds after discovery of change in condition, the FTO prompted the student to increase the oxygen to 15 L/min via nonrebreather and to lower the head of the stretcher.

The student quickly made the adjustments for oxygen and positioning of the patient after the FTO prompted him. The FTO documented as follows.

Change of Therapy   Changes course of treatment, within thirty (30) seconds, following change in patient's condition or presentation.

7. 1 ② 3 ++   (elapsed time: = 30)   you determined that there was no radial pulse, but you must act (at 30 sec. after "no radials") quickly to apply more oxygen and to place the patient supine

(Prompt:)   Differential Diagnosis   Knowledge of Protocols   (Implementation)

Notice that the FTO has documented that she gave the prompts at 30 seconds. She used quotation marks to indicate that she measured the 30 seconds from the time the student verbalized that radial pulses were absent. Notice also that she considered these prompts to be so important that this competency received an unsatisfactory score (2).

Remember that this unsatisfactory grade will result in an unsatisfactory overall score because this is a critical competency group.

Section 3   Overall Score: Satisfactory   ++   or   (Unsatisfactory)
(Instruction phase)   Were there... > 3 Prompts?   Have there been... > 3 Repetitive Prompts?

Scoring Professionalism and Affective Behavior

The patient is a 77-year-old female who complained of difficulty breathing. The student spoke to the patient in too loud a voice. The patient told the student "I am *not* hard of hearing." The FTO gave a hand signal to prompt the student to speak more quietly.

The student responded by saying, "I know what I'm doing." He continued to address the patient in a loud voice. The FTO took charge of patient care and apologized for the student's behavior. She then sent the student to the ambulance to set up equipment. The FTO documented student behavior, and her prompts, as follows:

Professional/Affective   Fulfills responsibilities for professional conduct and affective behavior as outlined in the *Manual for Students and FTOs*.

8. ① 2 3 ++   Do not assume that all geriatric patients are hard of hearing! Your comment that "I know what I'm doinig" was inappropriate ... see FTO comments section.

(Prompt:)   Honesty   (Courtesy)   Confidentiality   (Accepts Responsibility)   Accepts Constructive Criticism

Instructor Comments: Speaking too loudly will frequently offend patients. Making comments like "I know what I'm doing" is an inappropriate way to address the FTO. You must accept responsibility for your actions. You must learn how to avoid upsetting your patients. Had you followed my prompt you might have been able to finish the patient contact.

Notice that the FTO assigned this competency group an unsatisfactory score (1). This shows that the FTO considers this skill performance to be completely unsatisfactory. Remember that this competency group is considered a critical indicator of student performance (shaded in gray on the form). Students will also receive an unsatisfactory overall score whenever they receive an unsatisfactory score within a critical competency group.

Section 3	**Overall Score:**	Satisfactory	++	or	(Unsatisfactory)
(Instruction phase)		Were there... > 3 Prompts?			Have there been... > 3 Repetitive Prompts?

Scoring Performance of Psychomotor Skills

The patient is a 19-year-old male who was injured in a motor vehicle crash. The student performed several skills. Those skills that were performed correctly have been graded as satisfactory (3). The student received a prompt for c-spine immobilization. He was prompted to immobilize the thorax and legs before he immobilized the head. He received an unsatisfactory score (2) for that skill.

Remember that this competency group is not considered critical. An unsatisfactory score in this competency group does not have to result in an unsatisfactory overall score.

The Skill format (shown below) accommodates certain invasive skill procedures. Intravenous access and endotracheal intubation were included here to demonstrate how to score these skills.

Skill *Lung sounds*	**Skill** *O₂ via nonrebreather*	**Skill** *Spine board* (Immobilize) *head last*	
10. 1 2 ③ ++	1 2 ③ ++ (elapsed time: < 3 min.)	1 2 ③ ++	**Prompt:** *The risk of immobilizing the head first is that the (heavier) body will shift before it is secured. This could extend an injury!*
IV / ET Skill 1 2 ③ ++	S1 (S2) U1 U2		

The FTO documented the prompt for proper immobilization by circling the words *prompt* and *immobilize head last*. The FTO circled S2 to indicate that the student achieved IV access on his second attempt. All other skills received satisfactory scores (3). The student receives a satisfactory overall score.

Section 3	**Overall Score:**	(Satisfactory)	++	or	Unsatisfactory
(Instruction phase)		Were there... > 3 Prompts?			Have there been... > 3 Repetitive Prompts?

Scoring Radio or Phone Reports

Some agencies do not routinely call in reports to the receiving medical facility. Agencies that do not call in reports should remove this competency group from their critique forms.

The patient is a 28-year-old female who was involved in a high-speed motor vehicle crash. She was an unrestrained occupant and was ejected approximately 50 feet into a field of corn. The student was making a radio report to the trauma facility. All information given by the student was accurate, but the FTO reminded the student to include the mechanism of the injuries in the radio report. This competency group is not considered a critical indicator. The FTO has the option of not counting any prompts documented here.

Verbal Reports		(Radio)	Contacts medical control. Gives concise report and requests orders (PRN).
		(Transfer)	Gives complete report to appropriate staff member of receiving facility.
11. 1 ② 3 ++			include: speed of vehicle, "restrained," or "unrestrained," and ejection in radio report

Prompt:

Scoring the Verbal Report (Transfer of Care)

The patient is a 77-year-old female who presented with altered mental status. The patient was found on the tiled floor of a bathroom. The patient has a small hematoma on the occipital region of the skull. The student's verbal report focused on the possibility of a CVA. The FTO prompted the student to report the possibility that the change in mental status may be the result of a head injury. This is not a critical competency group.

Verbal Reports		(Radio)	Contacts medical control. Gives concise report and requests orders (PRN).
		(Transfer)	Gives complete report to appropriate staff member of receiving facility.
11. 1 ② 3 ++			the area of injury, and possible mechanism (ground level fall to hard surface) must be included in your report

Prompt:

Scoring the Written Report

The patient is a 21-year-old male who was involved in a motor vehicle crash. The student described the mechanism of the injuries in the narrative section of the report. Local standards recommend that this information be included in the History section of present illness. The FTO prompted the student to correct this error before completing the form.

Written Report		Provides complete documentation on Delaware patient care report form.
12. ① 2 3 ++		put mechanism of injury in HPI, not in narrative
		this is the fourth time I have prompted for this item

Prompt:

Notice that the FTO has scored this competency group as unsatisfactory (1). In this instance, the FTO has given this student the same prompt on three other occasions. This means that the student is receiving repetitive prompts on a certain skill.

The student must demonstrate the ability to learn from the FTO's prompts. Some students will not be able to change their performance even with multiple prompts from the FTO. These students should receive unsatisfactory overall scores beginning with the fourth patient contact, and the repetitive nature of the deficiency should be documented.

Students who require repetitive prompting are at risk for failure in the EMS education process. The student must demonstrate the ability to accept information from the FTO and use that information to improve performance.

Assigning an Overall Score

The preceding examples are for students who are in the instruction phase of the field internship. There is one important difference between scoring in the instruction phase and the evaluation phase. For purposes of demonstration only, during the instruction phase a student can receive as many as three prompts and still get a satisfactory overall score. One will be the maximum number for allowable prompts during the evaluation phase.

An FTO should expect that every student will require a substantial number of prompts early in the field internship process. Students who ultimately succeed will require fewer and fewer prompts as they gain more experience.

An FTO should also expect that most students will receive a large number of unsatisfactory overall scores early in the instruction phase. As students gain experience, they will require fewer prompts. A student's success rate for satisfactory overall scores will improve as the number of prompts decreases.

Recall that prompts documented in noncritical competency groups do not have to be counted (in total number of prompts) when computing an overall score. Skills and reports (radio, verbal, and written,) are examples of noncritical competency groups.

Let's look at an example of a patient contact where the student receives a satisfactory overall score: The patient is a 28-year-old female whose complaint was shortness of breath. The student was prompted four times by the FTO. The prompts were as follows:

- **Initial:** Prompt to apply oxygen after breathing was noted as "fast."
- **History:** Prompt to ask if the patient has a history of breathing problems.
- **Physical Exam:** Prompt to perform early lung sounds for respiratory patient.
- **Skills:** Prompt to identify coarse wheezes, when student said "rhonchi."

The FTO prompted the student four times on this patient contact. Three of these prompts were documented in a critical competency group. The fourth prompt was for performance of a physical skill (identifying coarse wheezes).

The FTO elected to count only those prompts that were documented in critical competency groups. Because only three prompts were counted, the FTO assigned a satisfactory overall score.

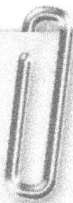

Section 3	Overall Score:	Satisfactory	++	or	Unsatisfactory
(Instruction phase)		Were there... > 3 Prompts?			Have there been... > 3 Repetitive Prompts?

However, remember that an FTO always has the option of including noncritical prompts in the overall score. If the FTO in this example elected to count all four prompts in the scoring process, the *overall score* would be recorded as follows:

Section 3	Overall Score:	Satisfactory	++	or	(Unsatisfactory)
(Instruction phase)		Were there...(> 3 Prompts?)			Have there been... > 3 Repetitive Prompts?

Repetitive prompts may result in unsatisfactory overall scores. The student is in the instruction phase. The overall score can be satisfactory even if the student receives three prompts. Assume that the patient is the same 28-year-old female from the previous example. The FTO gave only one prompt. She prompted the student to apply oxygen during the initial assessment. This was the fourth time this week that the FTO prompted the student to apply oxygen for a patient presenting with obvious signs of respiratory distress.

The standard of care for a patient who is short of breath includes timely administration of oxygen. The FTO has prompted this student to apply oxygen on four different patients. Obviously, this is the fourth repetitive prompt. The FTO documents the overall score as follows:

Section 3	Overall Score:	Satisfactory	++	or	(Unsatisfactory)
(Instruction phase)		Were there... > 3 Prompts?			(Have there been... > 3 Repetitive Prompts?)

Instructor Comments

The FTO uses this part of the critique form to make additional comments. This section can also be used to document a plan of action the student could use to improve his performance.

The patient is a 43-year-old male who presented in insulin shock. The patient was not able to fully protect his airway and had snoring respirations. The FTO prompted twice: She prompted the student to use a jaw thrust to open the airway. The FTO also prompted the student to apply better traction to the skin at the site of intravenous access. She elected to add the following comments.

Instructor Comments: (initial) Do not delay using jaw thrust for patients with snoring respirations. Call for an airway adjunct right away so that you will not be stuck holding the jaw for too long a time. (IV skill) You were holding traction directly below the IV site using your thumb. Try using your whole hand. Place your hand underneath the forearm below the site. Pull to the side, and down away from the elbow. This will keep your thumb out of the road of the catheter (eliminate possible contamination).

The student documents his response to the FTO. The student can also use this section to respond to The FTO's verbal feedback. For example:

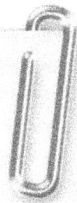

Student / Candidate Comments: __(initial) I believe that the FTO prompted before my 30 seconds of elapsed time__ __had passed. I think the FTO should have made this prompt a teaching point if she wanted me to act in less__ __than thirty seconds.   (IV skill) I appreciate the tip on another way to hold traction on the forearm.__

John 2. Student

The critique is signed and dated once all pertinent information has been entered. The FTO signs the critique form and gives it to the student. The student reviews the critique and enters any pertinent comments, as shown in the example. The student then signs the form. Either the student or the FTO can enter the date.

The FTO reminds the student that his signature is not an indication that he agrees with all of the FTO's documentation. The student's signature only indicates that he has had the opportunity to review the information on the critique form and make rebuttal comments.

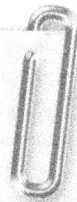

Instructor Signature: __Bob Q. FTO__   **Student Signature:** __Jon 2. Student__   **Date:** __10-11-03__

The following pages present two sample completed critique forms for a student in the instruction phase of the field internship. The first form is an example of a patient contact that received an unsatisfactory score. The second form is an example of a patient contact that received a satisfactory score.

| EMT-P Field Critique | Obs. | Rem. | TM | TL | TLE |

Circle each appropriate category: Pediatric (Geriatric) Trauma (Cardiac) Neuro (Respiratory) Gen. Med. Psych. OB

Section 1

Name: *John Doe*   Station: *Sta. 52*   Date: *5-21-03*

Instructor: *Jane Doe*   Run #: *1101*   Priority: (1) 1-M   2   3

Pt. age / sex: *68-F*   CC : *"she can't breathe" (by husband)*

Pt.'s Presentation, HPI, MOI: *somnolent—snoring respirations—cyanotic lips—P=126   BP=186/118   RR=36—history*

of COPD &CHF

Section 2   Score of: 1 = Unsatisfactory   2 = Unsatisfactory (parts satisfactory)   3 = Satisfactory

FTOs: *Circle both the word "Prompt" (and the skill that was prompted) to indicate that a prompt was given.*
Checkmark will indicate satisfactory skill performance.
Self-Test: Student's actions: Timely?   Appropriate?   Safe?   Within Protocol?

Scene / Multi-   Assesses scene safety, need for additional personnel, and takes appropriate actions. Document ability
to delegate, multitask, and make decisions here.

1. 1   2   (3)   ++   (elapsed scene time: 17 min.)   *must get IV started ASAP (before we can give NTG)*

(Prompt:) Safety   # of Patients/Personnel   Task Delegation (specify)   Multitasking   Decisions (where to . . . (when) to . . .)

Initial   Completes the initial assessment within thirty (30) seconds. Physically intervenes, within thirty (30)
seconds, to address problems found during the initial assessment.

2. 1   2   (3)   ++   (elapsed assessment time: *<30 sec*)   (elapsed intervention time: = 30 sec.)   *you described*
snoring—you must adjust the position of the head and neck

(Prompt:) c-spine   Airway / (Reposition) / Adjunct   Breathing / O_2 / BVM   Circulation / Flat / CPR   Disability (AVPU)   Expose

History   Obtains chief complaint, pertinent history of present illness, and pertinent past medical history.

3. 1   2   (3)   ++   Associated Symptoms: CP SOB IDDM H/A N / V / D   Recent: Trauma   Cough   Fever
delegated

Prompt: CC   HPI / PMH   Initial   (O, P, Q, R, S, T, A, M, P, L, E)   Hospital Preference   Other:

Physical Exam   Completes all pertinent components of physical examination.

4. 1   2   (3)   ++   Stroke Scale   Blood Sugar   Rapid Trauma Assessment

(Prompt:) P BP RR   Lung Sounds   Pupils   (Pulse Ox) $EtCO_2$ PMS   Edema   Palpate   Rhythm   (12 Lead)

Protocols/Standard/Care   Intervenes within the framework of accepted medical standards, protocols, and standing orders.
Student must begin appropriate treatment regimen within three (3) minutes.

5. 1   (2)   3   ++   (elapsed time: 3 min.)   *"Respiratory distress from COPD" was actually CHF.*

(Prompt:) (Differential Diagnosis)   Knowledge of Protocols   Implementation

Reassess	Reassesses, within five (5) minutes, for change in patient's condition or presentation.

6. 1   2   ③   ++   (elapsed time: <5 min.)

Prompt: CC   Initial   Vital Signs   Breath   Sounds   Pulse Ox   Pupils   PMS

Change of Therapy   Changes course of treatment, within thirty (30) seconds, following change in patient's condition or presentation.

7. 1   2   3   ++   (elapsed time:)   N/A

Prompt: Differential Diagnosis   Knowledge of Protocols   Implementation

---

Professional/Affective   Fulfills responsibilities for professional conduct and affective behavior as outlined in the *Manual for Paramedic Students and FTOs.*

8. 1   2   ③   ++

Prompt: Honesty   Courtesy   Confidentiality   Accepts Responsibility   Accepts Constructive Criticism

---

Communication   Establishes and maintains effective lines of communication.

9. 1   2   3   ++   Establishes Communication   Maintains Communication

Prompt: Patient   Family   Witness   EMS Personnel   Other Personnel

---

Skill lung sounds   "rhonchi" = rales   **Skill**   rhythm interpretation   sinus tach   **Skill**

10. 1   ②   3   ++   1   2   ③   ++   1   2   3   ++

   ⒾⓋ/ ET Skill   S1   Ⓢ2   (elapsed time: <3 min.)   Prompt:

   1   2   ③   ++   U1   U2

Verbal Reports   (Radio)   Contacts medical control. Gives concise report and requests orders (PRN).

      (Transfer)   Gives complete report to appropriate staff member of receiving facility.

11. 1   2   3   ++   N/A—delegated

Prompt:

Written Report   Provides complete documentation on Delaware patient care report form.

12. 1   2   ③   ++

Prompt:

Section 3   Overall Score: Satisfactory   ++   or   ⟨Unsatisfactory⟩

(Instruction phase)   Were there...⟨> 3 Prompts?⟩   Have there been... > 3 Repetitive Prompts?

Instructor Comments: *none*

_____

_____

Initial here if contact is "Unsatisfactory" based solely on severity of one prompt: _____   *Documentation is required.*

Student / Candidate Comments: *none*

_____

_____

_____

Instructor Signature: *Jane Doe*   Student Signature: *John 2. Doe*   Date: 5-21-03

EMT-P Field Critique

| Obs. | Rem. | TM | TL | TLE |

Circle each appropriate category: Pediatric Geriatric (Trauma) Cardiac (Neuro) Respiratory Gen. Med. Psych. OB

Section 1

Name: John Doe   Station: medic 17   Date: 5-30-03

Instructor: Jane Doe   Run #: 1213   Priority: (1) 1-M   2   3

Pt. age / sex: 19—M   CC : none—responds to physical stimulus only (altered mental status)

Pt.'s Presentation, HPI, MOI: AMS with mechanism for trauma—restrained driver—extrication

Obvious Right-femur FX–Hx of IDDM => Blood sugar=32   112—96/50—24 (clear lungs)

Section 2   Score of: 1 = Unsatisfactory   2 = Unsatisfactory (parts satisfactory)   3 = Satisfactory

FTOs: *Circle both the word "Prompt" (and the skill that was prompted) to indicate that a prompt was given.*
Checkmark will indicate satisfactory skill performance.
Self-Test: Student's actions: Timely?   Appropriate?   Safe?   Within Protocol?

Scene / Multi-   Assesses scene safety, need for additional personnel, and takes appropriate actions. Document ability
to delegate, multitask, and make decisions here.

1. 1   2   (3)   ++   (elapsed scene time: 8 min.)

Prompt: Safety✓   # of Patients/Personnel   Task Delegation (specify)✓   Multitasking✓   Decisions (where to . . . , when to . . .)✓

Initial   Completes the initial assessment within thirty (30) seconds. Physically intervenes, within thirty (30)
seconds, to address problems found during the initial assessment.

2. 1   2   (3)   ++   (elapsed assessment time: =30)   (elapsed intervention time: <30)

Prompt: c-spine   Airway / Reposition✓ / Adjunct   Breathing / O_2✓ / BVM   Circulation / Flat / CPR   Disability (AVPU)✓   Expose✓

History   Obtains chief complaint, pertinent history of present illness, and pertinent past medical history.

3. 1   2   3   ++   Associated Symptoms: CP SOB IDDM H/A N/V/D   Recent: Trauma Cough Fever
from passenger
Prompt: CC   HPI / PMH   Initial   (O, P, Q, R, S, T, A, M, P, L, E)   Hospital Preference   Other:

Physical Exam   Completes all pertinent components of physical examination.
inadvertent prompt (pupils) my partner took his penlight out, student saw him & proceeded to check pupils
4. 1   2   (3)   ++   Stroke Scale   Blood Sugar   Rapid Trauma Assessment
(Prompt:) P✓ BP (RR)   Lung Sounds✓   Pupils✓   Pulse Ox✓   EtCO$_2$ PMS✓   Edema   Palpate   Rhythm 12   Lead

Protocols/Standard/Care   Intervenes within the framework of accepted medical standards, protocols, and standing orders.
Student must begin appropriate treatment regimen within three (3) minutes.
5. 1   2   (3)   ++   (elapsed time: <3 min.)   trauma

Prompt: Differential Diagnosis   Knowledge of Protocols   Implementation

Revised 12-18-2005 by B. Nepon and B. Eberly

Reassess   Reassesses, within five (5) minutes, for change in patient's condition or presentation.

6. 1   2   (3)   ++   (elapsed time: <5 min.)

Prompt: CC ✓   Initial   Vital Signs ✓   Breath   Sounds ✓   Pulse Ox   Pupils ✓   PMS

Change of Therapy   Changes course of treatment, within thirty (30) seconds, following change in patient's condition
or presentation.

7. 1   2   3   ++   (elapsed time:)   N/A

Prompt: Differential Diagnosis   Knowledge of Protocols   Implementation

Professional/Affective   Fulfills responsibilities for professional conduct and affective behavior as outlined in the *Manual for
Paramedic Students and FTOs.*

8. 1   2   (3)   ++

Prompt: Honesty   Courtesy   Confidentiality   Accepts Responsibility   Accepts Constructive Criticism

Communication   Establishes and maintains effective lines of communication.

9. 1   2   3   ++   **Establishes Communication**   **Maintains Communication**

Prompt: Patient   Family   Witness   EMS Personnel   Other Personnel

Skill long back board   **Skill** rhythm   Sinus tach   **Skill** D—50 bolus
10. 1   2   (3)   ++   1   2   (3)   ++   1   2   (3)   ++
IV / ET Skill   S1   (S2)   (elapsed time: <3 min.)   Prompt:
1   2   (3)   ++   U1   U2

Verbal Reports   (Radio)   Contacts medical control. Gives concise report and requests orders (PRN).
(Transfer)   Gives complete report to appropriate staff member of receiving facility.

11. 1   2   (3)   ++

Prompt:

Written Report   Provides complete documentation on Delaware patient care report form.

12. 1   2   3   ++   N/A   written by FTO   wo were behind on reports

Prompt:

Section 3   Overall Score: (Satisfactory)   ++   or   Unsatisfactory
(Instruction phase)   Were there... > 3 Prompts?   Have there been... > 3 Repetitive Prompts?

Instructor Comments: *good contact—multiple problems—handled well*

Initial here if contact is "Unsatisfactory" based solely on severity of one prompt: *Documentation is required.*

Student / Candidate Comments: *thanks*

Instructor Signature: *Jane Doe*   Student Signature: *John 2. Doe*   Date: 5-30-03

In the Physical Exam competency group on the preceding critique form, the FTO notes the inadvertent prompt to check pupils. The reader should remember that inadvertent prompts are sometimes unavoidable. An FTO has to decide how much of an impact the inadvertent prompt had on the student's performance. In this example, the FTO elected not to count the inadvertent prompt.

When might an FTO count an inadvertent prompt? Most often, an FTO will count an inadvertent prompt if it is part of a repetitive pattern. For example, say that during the last two shifts the student has been prompted four times to apply oxygen to patients who were short of breath. The FTO's partner begins to open the oxygen bag. The student notices what the partner is doing and verbalizes that he wants oxygen applied to the patient. In this instance, the FTO would probably document the inadvertent prompt and score the Initial competency group as unsatisfactory.

This completes the chapter on scoring the instruction phase. The student's immediate goal is to complete the instruction phase and move on to the evaluation phase. The student's move to evaluation will depend on his EMS system's criteria.

This book does not establish rules for any EMS agency. One example of how completion criteria might be configured can be found in the Appendix A: *Manual for Paramedic Students and Instructors*. If the reader would like to view this example of completion criteria, they can review this information before continuing to the next chapter.

FTOTips ☑

Check your watch. If an inadvertent prompt occurs beyond a time limit, then count the prompt. Your partner, or another crew member, simply got to the prompt before you.

Check Your Knowledge

1. The student is in the instruction phase of the field internship. The FTO gave three prompts over the course of the patient contact. What should the student's overall score be?
   a. Satisfactory
   b. Unsatisfactory

   The correct answer is **a**. An FTO usually gives a satisfactory score when the student receives fewer than four prompts over the course of one patient contact.

2. The student is in the instruction phase of the field internship. The FTO gave three prompts over the course of the patient contact. The FTO also listed two other prompts as teaching points. What should the student's overall score be?
   a. Satisfactory
   b. Unsatisfactory

   The correct answer is **a**. Teaching points are not counted as prompts and are not included in the overall score. FTOs may document a prompt as a teaching point for a number of reasons. For example, an FTO may believe that the student has too little experience to perform a skill properly without help from the FTO (e.g., recognition of unusual lung sounds or use of certain medical history questions).

3. The competency for initial assessment and initial interventions is a critical competency group and is shaded in gray.
   a. True
   b. False

   The correct answer is **a**. Initial is considered a critical indicator of the student's ability to perform as a team leader. Students who are unable to find (and fix) problems related to the initial assessment will not be successful EMTs. All critical competency groups are shaded in gray.

4. The competency group for performance of physical skills is a critical indicator, and is shaded in gray.
   a. True
   b. False

   The correct answer is **b**. Psychomotor skills are not considered a critical indicator of the student's ability to perform as a team leader. It is not shaded in gray. Student performance of physical skills generally improves rapidly as the student gains experience. Students do not receive unsatisfactory overall scores because they had difficulty performing physical skills.

5. The FTO has given the same prompt on each of four separate patient contacts. The student will receive an unsatisfactory overall score for the fourth patient contact.
   a. True
   b. False

The correct answer is **a**. Repetitive prompting results in unsatisfactory overall scores. For example, say a student assessed four patients who were short of breath. The FTO prompted the student to apply oxygen during each of these patient contacts. This student is not learning from his mistakes. The fourth repetitive prompt should result in an unsatisfactory overall score, even if that is the only prompt for the entire patient contact.

Scoring the Evaluation Phase of the Field Internship

11

KEY POINTS

- Students usually require less prompting during the evaluation phase.
- One prompt or fewer results in a satisfactory overall score.
- Two or more prompts result in an unsatisfactory overall score.

This chapter explains how critique forms are used to document student performance during the evaluation phase of the field internship. As noted in the last chapter, critique forms offer the FTO a simple step-by-step format for writing evaluations of student performance.

This chapter provides additional examples of how critique forms are used to document student performance. This chapter also provides examples of scoring student performance during the evaluation phase of the field internship.

Students advance to the evaluation phase by demonstrating the ability to team-lead patient contacts. Students were successful in the instruction phase because they were able to team-lead patient contacts without too much assistance (prompts) from their FTOs.

During the instruction phase, the student was getting prompted too often if the patient contact required more than three prompts. Students should require less prompting from the FTO as their experience level increases.

A student will be given a satisfactory overall score when there is one prompt or no prompt. Throughout the evaluation phase of the field internship, students will receive unsatisfactory overall scores when the FTO prompts the student two or more times during one patient contact.

> **FTOTips** ☑
>
> The FTO may be worried that the student has been moved into the evaluation phase before he is ready. The student has only advanced because he has met the criteria for successful completion of the instruction phase. Holding him back risks getting the student too accustomed to the "three prompt cushion" afforded him in instruction.

Scoring in the Evaluation Phase

Example of an Unsatisfactory Overall Score

A student was prompted once in Initial and once in Physical Exam. Both of these competency groups are to be considered critical indicators of the student's team leadership ability. The FTO counts every prompt that is documented within a critical competency group. This student receives an unsatisfactory overall score because he received two prompts during one patient contact.

Remember that some competency groups are not considered critical. These unshaded competency groups measure performance of psychomotor skills. Prompts documented in these competency groups are usually not included in the overall score.

The FTO always has the option to count a noncritical prompt. Noncritical prompts are often counted when an FTO intervened to keep the student's actions from harming the patient or when these prompts are repetitive in nature.

The number of allowable prompts has decreased from three (during the instruction phase) to one (during the evaluation phase). As a result, the student's success rate is likely to decrease at the beginning of the evaluation phase. The student's success rate should increase dramatically as additional experience is gained.

Students who do not demonstrate an increasing success rate are at risk of failure in the evaluation process.

Documenting an Unsatisfactory Overall Score

The patient is a 48-year-old male who complained of substernal chest pain. He was alert and oriented at the time of the call. The patient was breathing rapidly. His skin was pale, wet, and cool to the touch.

The student began to obtain pertinent parts of the history and physical exam. He told the FTO that the patient is a high-priority patient. The student wanted to load the patient quickly and depart for the hospital. The FTO prompted the student to initiate oxygen therapy before loading the patient onto the stretcher. The FTO also prompted the student to get a complete list of medications before leaving the patient's residence.

All other performance was satisfactory.

The FTO scored the patient contact as follows:

Scene / Multi-   Assesses scene safety, need for additional personnel, and takes appropriate actions. Document ability to delegate, multitask, and make decisions here.

1.   1   2   ③   ++   (elapsed scene time: 11 min.)
apply oxygen before moving patient—movement will increase demand for O_2

(Prompt:) Safety   # of Patients/Personnel   Task Delegation (specify)   Multitasking   (Decisions)(where to ..., when to ...)

This is the first prompt for this patient contact. The FTO assigned a score of Satisfactory 3 (satisfactory with a prompt).

History   Obtains chief complaint, pertinent history of present illness, and pertinent past medical history.

3.   1   ②   3   ++   Associated Symptoms: CP   SOB   IDDM   H/A   N / V / D   Recent: Trauma   Cough   Fever
you must get a complete list of medications before we leave the patient's house

(Prompt:) CC   HPI / PMH   Initial   (O, P, Q, R, S, T, A,(M,)P, L, E)   Hospital Preference   Other:

The FTO scored History as Unsatisfactory 2 because this was the student's second prompt for this patient contact. Both Scene-Multi and History are considered critical indicators.

The entire patient contact receives an unsatisfactory grade whenever the student receives an unsatisfactory score (either 2 or 1) in a critical competency group.

Section 3	Overall Score:	Satisfactory	++	or	Unsatisfactory
(Instruction phase)		Were there... > 3 Prompts?		Have there been... > 3 Repetitive Prompts?	

An Unsatisfactory Overall Score with One Noncritical Prompt

The patient is a 71-year-old male who complained of chest pain. He was alert and oriented. He stated that his pain is "just like the time that he had his heart attack, a year and a half ago."

The patient's wife had given the patient a sublingual nitroglycerin tablet before the crew arrived. She had also applied a nitroglycerin patch to the patient's chest. The nitroglycerin is the wife's medication. The patient does not have a prescription for any nitroglycerin products. During transport to the hospital the patient complained of a sudden onset of "feeling weak and dizzy."

The student immediately checked for presence of a radial pulse. He found that there was no radial pulse. He immediately lowered the head of the stretcher and began to recheck the blood pressure. The FTO used a visual prompt to indicate that the student should remove the nitroglycerin paste from the patient's chest. The student removed the paste and resumed the recheck of the blood pressure. The FTO's comment "You already knew the blood pressure was low" refers to the absence of radial pulses as an indication of the patient's low blood pressure.

Change of Therapy   Changes course of treatment, within thirty (30) seconds, following change in patient's condition or presentation.

7. 1   2   3   ++   (elapsed time: = 30 sec.)
you adjusted the stretcher quickly after the patient lost radial pulses, remove the NTG paste ASAP!!! (you already knew BP was low)

Prompt: Differential Diagnosis   Knowledge of Protocols   Implementation

The student gave a radio report to the receiving hospital after he finished rechecking the blood pressure. The FTO prompted the student to include the patient's description of his chest pain in his report.

Verbal Reports   (Radio)   Contacts medical control. Gives concise report and requests orders (PRN).
(Transfer)   Gives complete report to appropriate staff member of receiving facility.

11. 1   ②   3   ++   *include patient's description "just like my last heart attack" this will be helpful to the hospital (and helpful to you, if you need to get orders . . .)*

Prompt:

In this instance, the FTO elects to count the noncritical prompt that was documented in the radio/phone report competency group. The FTO believes it is essential for the student to relay this information to the receiving hospital. This is also the second time the FTO has given the same prompt. The FTO counts this prompt and documents why this information is so important. The result is an unsatisfactory score.

Section 3 (Instruction phase)	Overall Score:	Satisfactory Were there... > 3 Prompts?	++	or	Unsatisfactory Have there been... > 3 Repetitive Prompts?

Another Option: The FTO Does Not Count the Noncritical Prompt

The FTO has the option of disregarding the prompt for radio/phone report. The radio report prompt does not have to be included in the total number of prompts for this patient contact. The FTO has this option because radio/phone reports is a noncritical indicator.

The FTO elects not to count the prompt for radio/phone report. This is the first time this type of prompt has been given to this student. The only "counted" prompt was documented in Change of Therapy. The student would receive a satisfactory overall score for the patient contact.

Change of Therapy   Changes course of treatment, within thirty (30) seconds, following change in patient's condition or presentation.

7. 1   2   3   ++   (elapsed time: = 30 sec.)
you adjusted the stretcher quickly after the patient lost radial pulses, remove the NTG paste ASAP!!! (you already knew BP was low)

(Prompt:)   Differential Diagnosis   Knowledge of Protocols   (Implementation)

Verbal Reports   (Radio)   Contacts medical control. Gives concise report and requests orders (PRN).
                       (Transfer)   Gives complete report to appropriate staff member of receiving facility.
11. 1   ②   3   ++   include patient's description "just like my last heart attack" this will be helpful to the hospital (and helpful to you, if you need to get orders . . .)

(Prompt:)

Section 3 (Instruction phase)	Overall Score:	Satisfactory Were there... > 3 Prompts?	++	or	Unsatisfactory Have there been... > 3 Repetitive Prompts?

Why did the FTO document the radio report prompt if it will not be recorded with the total number of prompts? There are two reasons this prompt should be documented:

- **The student uses this kind of feedback to improve performance.** The student is more likely to forget an FTO's advice if it is not documented on a critique form.
- **The FTO wants to know if the prompts have been effective, to see if the student can learn from his mistakes.** The FTO will know that the prompts have *not* been effective if the student keeps repeating the same mistake again and again. The FTO documents every prompt so trends in student performance can be monitored.

The FTO might elect to make the prompt a teaching point. Remember that there is no penalty for teaching points. They are not counted as prompts.

Essentially, a teaching point is the FTO's way of saying: "The radio report information was important! But, you were able to provide adequate patient care without describing the patient's pain in the radio report."

The FTO believes this information should be included in the radio report; however, she does not want to assign an unsatisfactory overall score to this patient contact. For that reason, the FTO elects to document the radio report prompt as a teaching point.

Change of Therapy   Changes course of treatment, within thirty (30) seconds, following change in patient's condition or presentation.

7. 1   2   (3)   ++   (elapsed time: = 30 sec.)   *you adjusted the stretcher quickly after the patient lost radial pulses, remove the NTG paste ASAP!!! you already knew the BP was low*

Prompt: Differential Diagnosis   Knowledge of Protocols   Implementation

Verbal Reports   (Radio)   Contacts medical control. Gives concise report and requests orders (PRN).
                          (Transfer)   Gives complete report to appropriate staff member of receiving facility.

11. 1   2   (3)   ++   *Teaching point—include the patient's description of his pain ("just like my last heart attack") in your report, this will be helpful to the hospital, and to you if you need to get orders, or a room assignment for the patient.*

Prompt:

In this example, the student would receive one prompt and one teaching point. The student would then receive a satisfactory overall score.

Section 3   Overall Score: Satisfactory   ++   or   Unsatisfactory
(Instruction phase)   Were there... > 3 Prompts?   Have there been... > 3 Repetitive Prompts?

The FTO Has Options

Why give the FTO so many options for documenting the same prompt? The reason is simple. The FTO is the on-scene evaluator. The FTO is in the best position to determine whether a student's actions were appropriate. The FTO is the best judge of student performance.

Each patient contact represents a unique set of circumstances. FTOs will evaluate each student performance based on the circumstances surrounding each patient contact.

FTOs need to have some latitude when evaluating student performance. This "room to maneuver" is an important part of this process of instruction and evaluation.

The FTO has latitude when scoring the patient contact: How much latitude does the FTO have? The FTO's self-test questions dictate how much maneuvering room is appropriate. The FTO can decide how much latitude to give the student by asking if the student's actions were:
- Safe?
- Timely?
- Appropriate?
- Within local protocol (standard of care)?

Look again at the maneuvering room that is built into the structure and function of the critique form:

- **Psychomotor skills are not considered critical.** FTOs do not usually count prompts that are documented in a noncritical competency group.
- **FTOs can make a prompt a teaching point.** This usually occurs when a prompt produces (history or physical exam) information that is not absolutely essential to care of the patient. FTOs use teaching points to give students the opportunity to learn the finer points of assessing and treating patients.

Remember these options. The student's percent success rate can be greatly affected by the FTO's use of these scoring options.

Example of a Satisfactory Overall Score

The patient is a 26-year-old female with a history of asthma. She complained of difficulty breathing. The patient actually used two one-word sentences to give this complaint ("Can't . . . breathe."). The student accurately described rapid breathing and presence of accessory muscle use.

The FTO gave one prompt for the entire patient contact. The student started to apply oxygen therapy with a nasal cannula. The FTO prompted the student to use a nonrebreather mask instead. The student applied the nonrebreather and completed the remainder of the patient contact satisfactorily.

The FTO documents this prompt in the Initial section.

Initial   Completes the initial assessment within thirty (30) seconds. Physically intervenes, within thirty (30) seconds, to address problems found during the initial assessment.

2. 1   2   ③   ++   (elapsed assessment time: = 30 sec.)   (elapsed intervention time: <30 sec.)

Use NRB for pt.'s who are breathing fast and can only use one-word sentences

(Prompt:)   c-spine   Airway / Reposition / Adjunct   Breathing ✓(O₂) BVM   Circulation / Flat / CPR   Disability (AVPU)   Expose ✗

All other competency groups were scored satisfactory 3 or N/A. The patient contact receives a satisfactory overall score because the student only needed one prompt from the FTO.

Section 3   Overall Score: (Satisfactory)   ++   or   **Unsatisfactory**

(Instruction phase)   Were there... > 3 Prompts?   Have there been... > 3 Repetitive Prompts?

What if this was a repetitive prompt? What if the FTO had prompted this student to use a nonrebreather four times this week?

Unsatisfactory Overall Score Because of Repetitive Prompting

The patient is a 26-year-old female with a history of asthma. She complained of difficulty breathing. The patient actually used two one-word sentences to give this complaint ("Can't . . . breathe."). The student accurately described rapid breathing and presence of accessory muscle use.

The FTO gave one prompt for the entire patient contact. The student started to apply oxygen therapy with a nasal cannula. The FTO prompted the student to use a nonrebreather mask instead. The student applied the nonrebreather and completed the remainder of the patient contact satisfactorily.

The FTO documents this prompt within initial assessment.

Initial   Completes the initial assessment within thirty (30) seconds. Physically intervenes, within thirty (30) seconds, to address problems found during the initial assessment.

2. 1 ② 3 ++   (elapsed assessment time: =30 sec.)   (elapsed intervention time: <30 sec.)

Use NRB for pt.'s who are breathing fast and can only use one-word sentences

Prompt: c-spine   Airway / Reposition / Adjunct   Breathing / O₂ / BVM   Circulation / Flat / CPR   Disability (AVPU)   Expose

This is the fourth time this week that the FTO has prompted the student to use high-flow oxygen on a patient who is severely short of breath.

This is an example of repetitive prompting. The FTO will enter the following overall score and document the repetitive problem as follows:

Section 3   **Overall Score:**   Satisfactory   ++   or   Unsatisfactory
(Instruction phase)   Were there... > 3 Prompts?   Have there been... > 3 Repetitive Prompts?

Instructor Comments: *This is the fourth time this week that I have prompted you to use a nonrebreather instead of a nasal cannula. Each of these patients has been severely short of breath. You must supply high-flow oxygen for unstable patients!*

This student has not been able to correct his mistakes. Students receiving more than three repetitive prompts should receive unsatisfactory overall scores on each subsequent prompt.

Unacceptable Scene Assessment and Poor Decision Making

The patient is a 61-year-old male who was involved in a motor vehicle crash. The crash involved only one vehicle. There is no evidence of significant mechanism. The patient was wearing a seatbelt, and the airbag did not deploy. The vehicle was still in gear and was resting against a tree upon EMS arrival. The engine was still running. The patient responds only to physical stimulus.

The student delegated c-spine control and began an initial assessment. The FTO gave two prompts. The FTO prompted the student to put the vehicle's transmission into the park position and to turn the ignition off. The FTO also prompted the student to check for medical alert tags. The FTO used this prompt to get the student to consider the possibility that a medical condition (i.e., insulin shock, CVA, cardiac event) might have caused the crash.

The student received three documented prompts even though the FTO only gave two verbal prompts. The FTO prompted the student to turn the vehicle off. She also prompted the student to look for medic alert tags.

The second prompt is documented in two places: in Scene-Multi and in the Physical Examination competency group. The single prompt (check for medical alert tags) serves two purposes. It addresses (1) whether the student can relate the lack of mechanism to the possibility of a medical condition and (2) whether the

FTOTips ☑

The reader may ask, "How can you grade a student who has never been in a similar patient contact before now?" As EMS providers, we encounter new types of patient contacts throughout our careers. What helps ensure that we provide safe, timely, appropriate care within local standards is that we have developed a routine—a method of assessing, decision-making, and treating—that helps us deal with the new and unknown. This process helps the student develop that routine.

student understands the importance of looking for evidence of a preexisting medical condition.

The FTO documents both prompts as follows. The FTO's written comments remind the student of what should be done in a situation like this.

Scene / Multi-   Assesses scene safety, need for additional personnel, and takes appropriate actions. Document abilityto delegate, multitask, and make decisions here.

1. 1   (2)   3   ++   (elapsed scene time: <10 min.)   (safety) put vehicle in park & turn off! (scene awareness/decisions) when to consider "medical problems" (with no apparent mechanism)

(Prompt:) (Safety)   # of Patients/Personnel   Task Delegation (specify)   Multitasking   Decisions (where to . . . , when to) . .)

Physical Exam   Completes all pertinent components of physical examination.

4. 1   (2)   3   ++   Stroke Scale   Blood Sugar   Rapid Trauma Assessment
Always check for medications/(medic alert tags) esp. with altered mental status

(Prompt:) P   BP   RR   Lung Sounds   Pupils   Pulse Ox   EtCO$_2$ PMS   Edema   Palpate   Rhythm   12 Lead

---

The student received three prompts. All other competency groups received satisfactory scores. The student receives an unsatisfactory overall score because he is in the evaluation phase and was prompted more than once.

Section 3   Overall Score: Satisfactory   ++   or   (Unsatisfactory)
(Instruction phase)   Were there... > 3 Prompts?   Have there been... > 3 Repetitive Prompts?

One Prompt = Satisfactory Overall Score

The patient is a 32-year-old female who said: "My heart feels like it's racing, and I'm really weak." The patient appeared pale and had no radial pulses.

The student's assessment and treatment was timely and appropriate. The FTO prompted once during the entire patient contact. The FTO wanted the student to find out (early in the patient contact) if the patient had ever had a similar episode before.

Why did the FTO give this prompt? The patient may know the nature of the medical condition. The patient may also know which treatments were effective the last time she experienced these symptoms. The FTO wants the students to learn the potential value of this kind of information.

History   Obtains chief complaint, pertinent history of present illness, and pertinent past medical history.

3. 1   2   (3)   ++   Associated Symptoms: CP   SOB   IDDM   H/A   N / V / D   Recent: Trauma   Cough   Fever
early check for previous similar episodes frequently helps with early diagnosis

(Prompt:) CC   HPI / PMH   Initial   (0, P, Q, R, S, T, A, M(P)L, E)   Hospital Preference   Other:

The student receives a satisfactory overall score because this was the only prompt given during this patient contact.

Section 3	**Overall Score:**	Satisfactory	++	or	Unsatisfactory
(Instruction phase)		Were there... > 3 Prompts?			Have there been... > 3 Repetitive Prompts?

Another Satisfactory Overall Score

The patient is a 57-year-old male who complained of chest pain that is "Just like my last heart attack." The patient's skin was pale, moist, and cool. Radial pulses were weak.

The student is in the evaluation phase. His protocol for treatment of cardiac-type chest pain includes giving sublingual nitroglycerin tablets and 1-inch of nitroglycerin paste. The protocol states that nitroglycerin should be withheld if the patient has taken an erectile dysfunction medication within the last 24 hours. When the student asked about erectile dysfunction drug use, the patient replied "Yes." The student then attempted to give the sublingual nitroglycerin. The FTO prompted the student to not give the medications.

Protocols/Standard/Care   Intervenes within the framework of accepted medical standards, protocols, and standing orders. Student must begin appropriate treatment regimen within three (3) minutes.

5.   1   2   ③   ++   (elapsed time: <3 min.)

you know the pt. had taken Viagra—NTG cannot be given—study protocols!

Prompt: Differential Diagnosis   Knowledge of Protocols   Implementation

This prompt was the only prompt for the patient contact. The student receives a satisfactory overall score.

Section 3	**Overall Score:**	Satisfactory	++	or	Unsatisfactory
(Instruction phase)		Were there... > 3 Prompts?			Have there been... > 3 Repetitive Prompts?

Methods for prompting do not change when the student moves from the instruction phase to the evaluation phase. The criteria for evaluating student performance *do* change. The student is expected to require less prompting during the evaluation phase of the field internship. Students demonstrate team leadership ability by needing fewer prompts from their FTOs.

Two samples of completed critique forms are shown on the following pages. The first critique is an example of a completed EMT-B form-evaluation phase. The second critique is an example of a completed EMT-P form-evaluation phase.

EMT-B Field Critique

Circle appropriate phrase: Observation   Instruction   (Evaluation)   *Submit for Review by Coordinator:*   Yes   (No)

Section 1

Student/Candidate: John Doe   Station: Sta. 13   Date: 6-21-03

FTO: Jane Doe   Incident #: 11238   Priority: 1   2   (3)

Pt. age / sex: 29—F   CC : "I can't breathe"

Pt.'s Presentation, HPI, MOI: alert/oriented—tachypneic—retractions—history of asthma—KNDA

          P=98   BP=132/78   RR=40—"worse than previous episodes ..."

Section 2   Score of: 1 = Unsatisfactory   2 = Unsatisfactory (parts satisfactory)   3 = Satisfactory

FTOs: *Circle the word "Prompt" (and the skill that was prompted) to indicate that a prompt was given.*
        Make a checkmark (through the skill) to indicate satisfactory performance of that skill.
FTO Self-test: Were the student's actions: Timely?   Appropriate?   Safe?   Within Protocol?

| **Scene / Multi-** | Assesses scene safety, need for additional personnel, and takes appropriate actions. Document ability to delegate, to multitask, and make decisions, here. |

1.   1   2   (3)   (elapsed scene time: 9 min.)

Prompt: Safety   # of Patients/Personnel   Task Delegation (specify)   multitasking   Decisions (where to . . . , when to . . .)

| **Initial** | Completes the initial assessment within thirty (30) seconds. Physically intervenes, within thirty (30) seconds, to address problems found during the initial assessment. |

2.   1   2   (3)   (elapsed assessment time: <30 sec.)   (elapsed intervention time: = 30 sec.)

(Prompt:) c-spine   Airway / Reposition / Adjunct   Breathing /(O₂)/ BVM   Circulation / Flat / CPR   Disability (AVPU)   Expose

| **History** | Obtains chief complaint, pertinent history of present illness, and pertinent past medical history. |

3.   1   (2)   3   Associated Symptoms: CP   SOB   IDDM   H/A   N / V / D   Recent: Trauma (Cough) (Fever)

(Prompt:) CC   HPI / PMH   Initial   (O, P, Q, R, S, T, A, M, P, L, E)   Hospital Preference   Other:

| **Physical Exam** | Completes all pertinent components of physical examination. |

4.   1   (2)   3   Stroke Scale   Blood Sugar   Rapid Trauma Assessment
                                    (to do lung sounds at 4 minutes)
(Prompt:) P   BP   RR   (Breath Sounds)   Pupils   Pulse Ox   PMS   Edema   Palpate   Other:

| **Protocols/Standard/Care** | Intervenes within the framework of accepted medical standards, protocols, and standing orders. EMT, or student, must begin appropriate treatment regimen within three (3) minutes. |

5.   1   2   (3)   (elapsed time: <3 min.)

Prompt: Knowledge of Protocols   Differential Diagnosis   Implementation

Prepared by B. Nepon and B. Eberly/Bayhealth Medical Center

Reassess   Reassesses, within five (5) minutes, for change in patient's condition or presentation.

6. 1 (2) 3 ++   (elapsed time: = 5 min.)

(Prompt:) (CC)   Initial   Vital Signs   Breath   Sounds   Pulse Ox   Pupils   PMS

Change of Therapy   Changes course of treatment, within thirty (30) seconds, following change in patient's condition or presentation.

7. 1 2 3   (elapsed time:)   N/A

Prompt: Knowledge of Protocols   Differential Diagnosis   Implementation

---

Professional/Affective   Fulfills responsibilities for professional conduct and affective behavior as outlined in the *Manual for Paramedic Students and FTOs*.

8. 1 2 (3) ++

Prompt: Honesty   Courtesy   Confidentiality   Accepts Responsibility   Accepts Constructive Criticism

---

Skill oxygen/nonrebreather   **Skill** lung sounds   **Skill** Decreased bases/wheezes at apices

9. 1 2 (3)   1 2 (3)   1 2 3

Skill

1 2 3   Prompt:

Verbal Reports   Gives complete report to appropriate staff member of receiving facility.

10. 1 2 (3)

Prompt:

Written Report   Provides complete documentation on Delaware patient care report form.

11. 1 2 (3)

Prompt:

Section 3   Overall Score: Satisfactory   ++   or   (Unsatisfactory)

(Instruction phase)   Were there... > 3 Prompts?   Have there been... > 3 Repetitive Prompts?

FTO Comments: *give oxygen ASAP to people breathing at 40/min.*

Student / Candidate Comments: OK—J.D.

Instructor Signature: *Jane Doe*   Student Signature: *John Doe*   Date: 6-21-03

EMT-P Field Critique	Obs.	Rem.	TM	TL	TLE

Circle each appropriate category: Pediatric (Geriatric) Trauma (Cardiac) Neuro Respiratory Gen. Med. Psych. OB

Section 1

Name: *John Doe*   Station: *Medic 38*   Date: *6-22-03*

Instructor: *Jane Doe*   Run #: *10179*   Priority: (1) 1-M   2   3

Pt. age / sex: *67—M*   CC : *"my chest hurts" and "I'm a little short of breath"*

Pt.'s Presentation, HPI, MOI: *alert/oriented—pale, moist, cool, skin—noreproducible pain*

Similar to last heart attack—108—162/84—24—with basilar rales

Section 2   Score of: 1 = Unsatisfactory   2 = Unsatisfactory (parts satisfactory)   3 = Satisfactory

FTOs: *Circle both the word "Prompt" (and the skill that was prompted) to indicate that a prompt was given.*
Checkmark will indicate satisfactory skill performance.
Self-Test: Student's actions: Timely?   Appropriate?   Safe?   Within Protocol?

Scene / Multi-
Assesses scene safety, need for additional personnel, and takes appropriate actions. Document ability to delegate, multitask, and make decisions here.

1.   1   2   (3)   ++   (elapsed scene time: *10 min*)

Prompt: Safety   # of Patients/Personnel   Task Delegation (specify)   multitasking   Decisions (where to . . . , when to . . .)

Initial
Completes the initial assessment within thirty (30) seconds. Physically intervenes, within thirty (30) seconds, to address problems found during the initial assessment.

2.   1   2   (3)   ++   (elapsed assessment time: *<30*)   (elapsed intervention time: *<30*)

Prompt: c-spine   Airway / Reposition / Adjunct   Breathing / O_2 / BVM   Circulation / Flat / CPR   Disability (AVPU)   Expose

History
Obtains chief complaint, pertinent history of present illness, and pertinent past medical history.

3.   1   2   (3)   ++   Associated Symptoms: CP   SOB   IDDM   H/A   N / V / D   Recent: Trauma   Cough   Fever

Prompt: CC   HPI / PMH   Initial   (O, P, Q, R, S, T, A, M, P, L, E)   Hospital Preference   Other:

Physical Exam
Completes all pertinent components of physical examination.

4.   1   2   (3)   ++   Stroke Scale   Blood Sugar   Rapid Trauma Assessment

Prompt: P   BP   RR   Lung Sounds   Pupils   Pulse Ox $EtCO_2$ PMS   Edema   Palpate   Rhythm 12 Lead

Protocols/Standard/Care
Intervenes within the framework of accepted medical standards, protocols, and standing orders. Student must begin appropriate treatment regimen within three (3) minutes.

5.   1   2   (3)   ++   (elapsed time: *<3 min.*)

Prompt: Differential Diagnosis   Knowledge of Protocols   Implementation

Revised 12-18-2005 by B. Nepon and B. Eberly

Reassess   Reassesses, within five (5) minutes, for change in patient's condition or presentation.

6. 1   2   ③   ++   (elapsed time: = 5 min.)

Prompt: CC   Initial   Vital Signs   Breath   Sounds   Pulse Ox   Pupils   PMS

Change of Therapy   Changes course of treatment, within thirty (30) seconds, following change in patient's condition or presentation.

7. 1   2   3   ++   (elapsed time:)   N/A

Prompt: Differential Diagnosis   Knowledge of Protocols   Implementation

Professional/Affective   Fulfills responsibilities for professional conduct and affective behavior as outlined in the *Manual for Paramedic Students and FTOs*.

8. 1   2   ③   ++

Prompt: Honesty   Courtesy   Confidentiality   Accepts Responsibility   Accepts Constructive Criticism

Communication   Establishes and maintains effective lines of communication.

9. 1   2   3   ++   Establishes Communication   Maintains Communication

Prompt: Patient   Family   Witness   EMS Personnel   Other Personnel

Skill lung sounds "Basilar rales"   **Skill** rhythm interpretation   **Skill** "sinus rhythm/PVC's"

10. 1   2   ③   ++   1   2   ③   ++   1   2   ③   ++

(IV)/ ET Skill   S1   (S2)   (elapsed time: <3 min.)   **Prompt:** Keep your thumb out of the way! Second time was better!

1   ②   3   ++   U1   U2

Verbal Reports   (Radio)   Contacts medical control. Gives concise report and requests orders (PRN).
(Transfer)   Gives complete report to appropriate staff member of receiving facility.

11. 1   2   ③   ++   N/A done by FTO

Prompt:

Written Report   Provides complete documentation on Delaware patient care report form.

12. 1   2   ③   ++

Prompt:

Section 3   Overall Score: (Satisfactory)   ++   or   Unsatisfactory
(Instruction phase)   Were there... > 3 Prompts?   Have there been... > 3 Repetitive Prompts?

Instructor Comments: _did not count IV prompt (noncritical)/J.D_

Initial here if contact is "Unsatisfactory" based solely on severity of one prompt: _Documentation is required._

Student / Candidate Comments: _thanks for the tip on the IV!/J.D._

Instructor Signature: _Jane Doe_   Student Signature: _John Doe_   Date: _6-22-03_

Check Your Knowledge

1. The student is in the evaluation phase of the field internship. The FTO gave three prompts over the course of the patient contact. What would the student's overall score be?
   a. Satisfactory
   b. Unsatisfactory

   The correct answer is b. During the evaluation phase of the field internship, the student receives an unsatisfactory overall score if he gets more than one prompt. Students who have completed the instruction phase should require less prompting from the FTO.

2. The student is in the evaluation phase of the field internship. The FTO gave one prompt over the course of the patient contact. The FTO also listed one other prompt as a teaching point. What would the student's overall score be?
   a. Satisfactory
   b. Unsatisfactory

   The correct answer is a. Teaching points do not count as prompts. An FTO will document a teaching point whenever a prompt was more of a "good to know" point and not something the student absolutely needed to provide adequate patient care.

3. The student is in the evaluation phase of the field internship. The FTO gave two prompts in the Initial competency group. This is a critical indicator. What would the student's overall score be?
   a. Satisfactory
   b. Unsatisfactory

   The correct answer is b. The student received two prompts. Both prompts are counted even though they are documented in the same competency group. That competency group is scored as an unsatisfactory 2 or 1. The patient contact is also assigned an unsatisfactory overall score.

4. The student is in the evaluation phase of the field internship. The FTO gave one prompt in radio/phone reports. The FTO also gave a prompt in written reports. Neither of these competency groups is considered a critical indicator of team-leadership performance. No prompts were repetitive. What would the student's overall score be?
   a. Satisfactory
   b. Unsatisfactory

   The correct answer is a. Prompts documented in noncritical competencies are not usually counted. However, an FTO may elect to count these prompts if (1) the prompt is a repetitive prompt or (2) the prompt was necessary to keep the student from harming the patient.

5. The FTO prompted the student to take a radial pulse rate (physical exam). The student does not agree with his FTO. The student contends that he took the pulse rate and reported it to the FTO. What should the student do?

a. Say nothing to the FTO, he doesn't want the FTO mad at him.

b. Document his opinion in the Student Comments section.

c. Call and complain to the program coordinator.

d. Both a and c

The correct answer is **b**. The critique form has space set aside for both parties to enter comments. Students address differences of opinion by writing responses to the FTO within the Student Comments section. FTOs should periodically remind students to document their concerns or differences of opinion. No student complaint should be considered valid unless it is supported by timely documentation.

12

A Day in the Life of a Field Training Officer

KEY POINTS

- Both the FTO and student must utilize time effectively between patient contacts.
- The FTO must give prompt verbal feedback after every call.
- The FTO must complete paperwork quickly so that the student has no (late) surprises.
- The FTO must continue to give the student positive reinforcement and context to reduce undue stress.

No single book could provide an FTO with the right answers for every conceivable question, because too many sets of challenging circumstances are likely to arise. However, an FTO should be able to handle most of the challenges that will arise by using the tips and techniques in this book.

The FTO provides effective instruction by giving real-time prompts to the student. These prompts motivate the student to do the right thing. Time limits motivate the FTO to offer a prompt at a particular point in time, thereby teaching the student the right time to perform a particular skill.

The patient benefits from having the correct assessment and treatment skills performed at the right time. Once the patient contact has been completed, the FTO documents each prompt that was given to the student. This documentation provides a written record of the student's performance. It also provides a written record of how, and when, the FTO provided instruction to the student.

For these reasons, the three most important tools for the FTO are:

1. Prompts
2. Time limits
3. Documentation

The following scenario describes a day in the life of a fictitious FTO. It seems fitting to end this book with a representation of a typical day's work for one FTO.

Beth is the FTO for a municipal paramedic service. Paramedic units within this system are staffed by two paramedics who work two 10-hour day shifts followed by two 14-hour night shifts. Day shifts begin at 0800 hours and end at 1800 hours.

Beth and her partner Ken staff Medic 77, a nontransport chase vehicle. Patient transport is accomplished in ambulances staffed by EMT-Basic providers. Stable patients are transported to the hospital accompanied by only one of Medic 77's paramedics. Unstable patients are accompanied by both of Medic 77's paramedics. Transport time varies from 2 to 20 minutes. Employee compensation is adequate and, at this point in time, many of this EMS service's providers view themselves as career professionals.

Sam is a paramedic student who has been employed and sent to school by the same agency that employs Beth. He is entering the 12th month of his paramedic education offered by a community college. He is beginning the third week of a 12-week field internship and is in the second week of the instruction phase.

The following is a rundown of a typical day for Medic 77's paramedics and student.

0726   Beth arrives at the station and begins to assemble protective gear, forms, and the notebooks she will need to document student performance.

0733   Sam arrives and Beth notes his arrival time on the *FTO Checklist* for this shift. She also notes that Sam is properly attired and has the required equipment. Sam arrived at 0752 (7 minutes past his designated arrival time) for his first shift with Beth two weeks ago. He does not want his tardiness documented a second time.

0741   Under Beth's supervision, Sam begins the equipment check. Ken arrives and begins checking the vehicle.

0750   Sam relates that the cardiac monitor is low on paper. Beth procures the paper and guides Sam through the replacement process.

0755   Shift change is accomplished with the off-going shift indicating that all equipment is present and functioning.

0801   Medic 77 leaves the station and proceeds toward a local coffee shop. While en route, Beth asks Sam if he has any questions concerning last week's calls or questions about last week's paperwork. Sam says that he thought the last patient contact, from the last night shift, should have been scored satisfactory instead of unsatisfactory. Beth says, "You had four prompts on that call. That's one too many. Also, if you disagreed with me, you should have told me right away and then written your comments on the critique form before you signed it."

0819   Just after coffee was acquired, Medic 77 received a call for a 41-year-old male with chest pain at a large credit card company's office. Sam says, "It's probably musculoskeletal." Ken replies, "Don't bet on it. We see a fair number of stress-related MIs come out of that building."

0826   Medic 77 makes contact with the patient. Assessment and treatment are provided in accordance with local ACS protocol. Beth and Sam accompany the patient to hospital.

0842   Transfer of care is completed at the medical facility. Ken was called to a motor vehicle crash (MVC), so Beth assigns Sam to work on the patient care report while she restocks equipment. She then splits her time between completing a critique form for this contact and making suggestions to Sam as he works his way through the PCR. She talks about the contact as she completes the critique: "I prompted at 30 seconds for oxygen, prompted for multitasking (do simultaneous history questions and vital signs), prompted to start an IV before nitroglycerin administration. I also prompted you to note basilar rales during lung sounds. Counting last week, that is the third time you have missed fine rales on a cardiac patient. There were four prompts, so the contact is an unsatisfactory."

0855   Sam is more quiet than usual, so Beth asks if anything is wrong. Sam says, "I thought I was going to do better than this." Beth says, "Listen, this is not unusual this early in the internship. You just came back from four days off. We see this frequently. Students often lose a little ground when they come back from their days off. You should expect to get better throughout the day and throughout the field internship." Beth then lists a number of things that Sam did well during the contact. The positive reinforcement seems to improve his attitude.

0915   Ken arrives and restock is completed. Medic 77 goes en route back into their district.

0920   Medic 77 responds to an MVC that is reported as a rollover with ejection involving three patients. Two units and the field supervisor are responding.

0926   Both medic units arrive. Medic 77 is closest to two of the patients and begins assessment and treatment. The supervisor arrives and immediately calls Beth's attention to Sam's lack of a turnout coat. Sam dons the coat and resumes care. Beth gives prompts for task delegation (BLS to bring additional equipment) and for reassessing the blood pressure when Sam's patient became very pale and complained of dizziness.

1011   Transport and transfer of care has been completed for all patients. Ken is restocking while Sam writes the PCR and Beth writes the critique. Sam says, "I guess I am going to get an 'unsat' because I forgot my gear." Beth says: "No. You only had two prompts (delegation and a repeat blood pressure). The prompt from the supervisor doesn't count. I am responsible for your safety and for your actions. If I don't give the prompt first, then it becomes my responsibility. I will document the need for turnout gear on the critique form, not as a prompt, but as a teaching point."

1033   Medic 77 clears the hospital and responds to headquarters where the supervisor and Beth discuss her responsibilities with regard to the student.

1100   Medic 77 goes en route to coffee shop, acquires beverages, and then returns to station. Sam states that he feels like he has gotten Beth in trouble. She replies, "Being an FTO is sometimes challenging, especially when several things are happening at once. I am responsible for both my actions and your actions. It is almost impossible to track everything that is going on 100% of the time, but that's my responsibility. I cannot hold you accountable for something that I missed. However, you should expect that I will not miss it again, and that you will be accountable if it does happen again."

1138   Medic 77 stops to pick up an early lunch and returns to the station. While eating, Beth says to Sam, "I haven't seen you carrying any textbooks. Have you started studying for the written Registry exam yet?" Sam replies, "No, our instructors at the school told us that we would prepare for the Registry exams after the field internship was completed." Beth comments, "You should consider bringing a couple of books, specifically your text, in case you need to review material related to a patient contact and a study guide that helps prepare you for the written exam. By the time you reach the end of field internship, you will be ahead of the game, as long as you use your down time (in between calls) wisely."

1247   Medic 77 responds to a call for a 66-year-old female with difficulty breathing. Once on scene at 1256, Sam begins to assess and treat the patient. The patient has a 10-year history of insulin-dependent diabetes mellitus and no history of respiratory problems. Lung sounds are clear. Sam says he is going to run a 12-lead cardiogram to rule out an atypical cardiac presentation. Subsequently, Sam prints out a 3-lead monitor strip. Beth glances at it and asks, "What do you see on the 12-lead?" Sam discovers that he has run only a 3-lead and prints another strip. Beth glances again and says, "That's another 3-lead." At this point, Tom (an EMT-B on the transport unit) reaches toward the monitor to push the correct button for a 12-lead printout. Sam snatches the machine away from Tom and says, "I have to learn how to do this myself!" Beth quietly tells Sam, "That's enough." She then looks at Tom, shows him a stop sign (palm of hand), and puts her finger to her lips, silently asking Tom to let it go, for now.

FTOTips ☑

The FTO must remind the student that he is not expected to be perfect. Comments from the FTO after a patient contact are not counted as prompts in the grading process. These comments are for enrichment, or to cover an item that the FTO did not get to during patient care.

FTOTips ☑

Use down time effectively. The student can be studying for exams. The FTO and student could be practicing scenarios to iron out rough spots seen during patient contacts. They can review a piece of new equipment.

1317   Medic 77 completes transfer of care for their 66-year-old AMI patient. Ken starts restocking supplies, while Sam begins writing the PCR. Beth confers privately with Tom. She thanks him for not getting into a verbal exchange (with Sam) on scene and asks that he stick around for a few minutes. Beth then approaches Sam and takes him outside where they can have a private conversation. Beth says, "Your patient assessment and your subsequent treatment choices were appropriate for this patient. I gave no prompts related to those areas. Unfortunately, your interaction with Tom was completely inappropriate. I am scoring the contact unsatisfactory based on that single prompt, which will be documented in the affective behavior competency group." Sam complains, "Tom and I have had issues before." Beth says, "Don't go there! You are required to demonstrate professional behavior, especially when you are with a patient. The last thing a 66-year-old lady who is having a heart attack wants is to be in the middle of an argument. *And*, I will not listen to excuses. Whatever happened between you and Tom in the past has no bearing on today's issues. The excuse will be documented as a second prompt. You will now go and apologize to Tom. We will talk more about this call after I have completed the critique."

1407   Medic 77 clears the hospital and goes en route to a call for a 13-year-old female whose complaint is shortness of breath secondary to asthma. During the contact, Beth prompts Sam to begin setting up for the IV while he is asking history questions (multitasking).

1430   Following transfer of care, Sam privately asks Beth why she prompted him to begin setting up the IV equipment so early in the call. Beth says, "There were two reasons for that prompt: One is that your protocol includes use of intravenous steroids. Establishing early IV access allows you to administer the medication at an earlier point in time. The second reason for the prompt was that you still need to improve your multitasking skills. In this case, you should be getting a medical history at the same time you are assembling equipment. You must learn to be an effective time manager. This contact will be scored as satisfactory with two prompts."

1517   Medic 77 returns to station. Following a short break, Beth begins questioning Sam about their EMS system's standing orders. She is probing to see if there are any gaps in his knowledge of their local treatment protocols. At the same time, Beth demonstrates multitasking by putting the finishing touches on the critique forms for today's patient contacts.

1550   Ken invites Sam to help him wash the unit. Beth says Sam can help in a few minutes, after she and Sam review the critiques and sign the forms.

1640   Medic 77 responds to an MVC in a mall parking lot. There was a report of vehicle rollover.

1646   The transport unit arrives on scene and relays message that there was no rollover and that there are no patients requiring treatment. Medic 77 is advised to cancel their response.

1654   Medic 77 is in quarters. Beth asks Sam if he has any questions about today's patient contacts or questions about any of the prompts he received today. Sam says, "No, I understand what each of the prompts was for." Beth then says, "There are two things I want to mention. First, you must learn to control what you say, and what you do, when you are on scene. Good rapport between providers is an essential part of this business. Second, I gave two prompts today for multitasking. You have at least three prompts for multitasking counting last week. This is now a repetitive prompt situation. Any additional prompts for multitasking will result in an automatic unsat score for that patient contact."

1728   Medic 77's on-coming crew arrives, and relieves the day crew.

1730   Beth advises Sam, "Remember that you are not expected to perform like an experienced provider at this point in the field internship. If you have any questions, you should ask them. I suggest you make a note on the back of your gloves just before we go on scene. Just write 'multitask.' Then when you are working, you can glance at the note and it will remind you to 'talk-and-do.'" Beth is completing the both the *Daily* (run) *Log* and the daily *FTO Checklist* as she conducts this discussion. At 1752 Beth makes sure all of the day shift's gear has been removed from the unit and then escorts Sam from the station. Her shift as an FTO is complete.

Check Your Knowledge

1. The student is responsible for everything that occurs during the patient contact.
   a. True
   b. False

The correct answer is **b**. False. The FTO is ultimately responsible for all that happens during the patient contact. The student is responsible for entry-level performance.

2. The student's time is his own between patient contacts.
   a. True
   b. False

The correct answer is **b**. False. The FTO and student must make good use of available down time, within reason. We all need to catch our breath sometimes; however, written protocols and texts can be studied, equipment can be reviewed, and scenarios can be conducted.

Manual for Paramedic Students and Instructors

A

This document includes the following:
- Criteria for successful completion of the clinical and field internship semesters
- Performance guidelines for paramedic students and paramedic instructors

Prepared by Bruce A. Nepon and Barry R. Eberly
EMS Education Department of Bayhealth Medical Center, Dover, Delaware
Revised and edited by the Paramedic Technology Program Faculty DTCC

Table of Contents

PART 1: For Students and Instructors

Purpose, Goal, and Objectives

Purpose

This manual describes the techniques that paramedic instructors will use when instructing and evaluating paramedic students and the criteria students must fulfill to successfully complete each of the internship semesters. The purpose of this manual is twofold. First, the manual establishes guidelines (rules of conduct) for both students and instructors. Second, it serves as a reference document that contains the answers to many frequently asked questions.

Goal

Paramedic students must fulfill the requirements outlined in this manual in order to successfully complete their clinical and field semesters. Paramedic instructors are expected to follow the guidelines set forth in this document whenever they provide instruction and evaluation to students. The goal is to establish performance expectations (of both instructors and students) that present a comprehensive educational opportunity to every paramedic student.

Objectives

Students and instructors should use information contained in this manual to help them to understand:
- Terminology that is unique to this process of instruction and evaluation
- The criteria for satisfactory performance of various paramedic skills
- The techniques used to document student skill performance
- The criteria for satisfactory (overall score) management of a patient contact
- The criteria for successful completion of both clinical and field semesters

Overview

The method presented for teaching and evaluating paramedic students is designed to be consistent from course to course and from semester to semester. Instructors use the same methods of instruction and evaluation during (1) patient assessment laboratory courses, (2) the clinical internship semester, and (3) the field internship semester.

The criteria for successful completion of the clinical and field internships are defined in Section 2 of this manual. Students who fulfill these criteria will successfully complete the clinical and field internship semesters.

A student will sometimes require prompts during a patient contact. These prompts are documented on a critique form. The assigned instructor monitors the number(s) and type(s) of prompts given throughout the course of the clinical and field semesters. A student who consistently requires an excessive amount of prompting will not successfully complete the semester.

Remediation will be considered for a student who is not meeting the criteria for successful completion of any portion of the clinical or field internships.

Refer to Section 2 for more detailed information regarding criteria for successful completion of the clinical and field internships.

Definitions

clinical   Hospital environment.

clinical internship   Portion of instruction and evaluation of paramedic students that is devoted to patient care in the hospital environment. Students may be assigned to paramedic units during this semester at the discretion of the program coordinator.

competency   A group of related skills. The various competencies are found in Section 2 of the Critique Form.

critical competency   A competency that is considered "critical" to the student's ability to manage patient care. These competencies are shaded gray on the Critique Form.

Critique Form   Form used to document student performance.

Daily Log   Envelope with preprinted form that logs the student's activities and secures all clinical paperwork for the assigned rotations.

delegation   The assignment of a task to a team member and the subsequent monitoring that the task is completed in a timely and safe manner.

differential diagnosis   The identification of probable diseases or conditions based on patient history, assessment, and physical examination; also known as a *field impression*.

field   Prehospital environment.

field internship   Portion of instruction and evaluation of paramedic students that is devoted to patient care in the prehospital environment.

Manual for Paramedic Students and Instructors   Document that defines the performance requirements for students and instructors.

FTO   Field Training Officer.

multifarious   A patient presentation that consists of a number of different and disparate signs and symptoms or that requires treatment under multiple pathways.

multitask   The concurrent operation of two or more processes by one person.

OEMS   Office of Emergency Medical Services.

paramedic instructor   A person who provides didactic or clinical instruction for paramedic students or an FTO who teaches and evaluates paramedic students in the prehospital environment.

paramedic student   Student enrolled in the paramedic technology program.

Priority One (1)   A patient suffering from an immediate life- or limb-threatening injury or illness.

Priority One-M (1-M)   A patient suffering from an immediate, *multifarious*, life- or limb-threatening injury or illness.

Priority Two (2)   A patient suffering from a potentially life- or limb-threatening injury or illness.

Priority Three (3)   A patient suffering from an injury or illness that requires medical attention but does not immediately, or potentially, threaten life or limb.

Program Coordinator   Person in charge of the paramedic program for Delaware Technical and Community College.

prompt   Stimulus used by an instructor to improve, or correct, a student's performance.

questionnaire   Form used by students to evaluate instructor performance. Student may also use this form submit questions or suggestions related to the educational program.

satisfactory   A skill performance that is within acceptable parameters.

Standing Orders Test   A required test that is given by an authorized agent of the OEMS designed to measure a paramedic's knowledge of the standing orders.

teaching point   Information important to patient care that is beyond the student's expected level of competency or a prompt from paramedic instructor that was not given in a timely manner.

Team Member (TM)   Student being evaluated only on the performance of individual skills.

Team Leader (TL)   Student responsible for managing patient care (instruction phase).

Team Leader Evaluated (TLE)   Student responsible for managing patient care (evaluation phase).

unsatisfactory   A skill performance that is not within acceptable parameters. Documentation must include a specific explanation of unsatisfactory performance.

Description of Clinical Critique Form by Section

Section 1: Required Information

1.1 Patient Category

1.2 Student Name

1.3 Department

1.4 Date Patient Was Assessed

1.5 Instructor Name

1.6 Priority of Patient (Priority 1, 1-M, 2, or 3)

1.7 Patient Age and Sex

1.8 Patient's Chief Complaint

1.9 Patient's Presentation (include pertinent mechanism of injury and/or history of present illness)

Section 2: Scoring of Competency Indicators

- Score of 3 indicates satisfactory performance of a competency indicator.
  - ++ indicates exceptional performance (beyond entry-level provider) of a competency indicator.
- Score of 2 indicates unsatisfactory performance of a competency indicator, although parts of the competency were performed satisfactorily.
- Score of 1 indicates unsatisfactory performance of a competency indicator.
- Each competency has space for an explanation of unsatisfactory performance. Students should refer to an instructor's "comments" when developing an action plan.

Elapsed time: Certain competencies have space allotted for documentation of elapsed time. Failure to complete a skill or competency within the specified time frame may be cause for the student to receive an unsatisfactory score.

2.1 Scene/Multiscene

Scene management includes scene safety, need for triage, and coordination of resources. The student will be required to delegate tasks. The student will be required to perform skills. Skill performance often must be accomplished simultaneously with task delegation and history-gathering. This skill is referred to as "multitasking."

2.2 Initial (Assessment and Treatment)

The student must complete the initial assessment and manage the patient appropriately. Refer to the Critique Form for time limits and interventions related to the initial assessment.

2.3 History

History includes patient's chief complaint (CC), history of present illness (HPI), and past medical history (PMH). The student must gather all pertinent information, relative to the patient's complaint or presentation.

2.4 Physical Exam

The student must complete a physical examination on each patient. This exam will include all pertinent exam procedures indicated by the patient's complaint or presentation. A list of prompt items for commonly used exam procedures is included in the Critique Form.

2.5 Protocols/Standard of Care

The patient must receive treatment that is in accordance with the local standard of care. The acceptable standard of care is outlined in the *State of Delaware Paramedic Standing Orders*.

2.6 Reassess

Change in the patient's condition may result from interventions or continuation of a disease, or injury, process. The student must reassess the patient for change in condition. Some changes in condition occur quickly. The student will be required to reassess in fewer than 5 minutes whenever there is a precipitous change in patient condition.

2.7 Change of Therapy

Change in the patient's condition may require change in therapy. The student must implement, or delegate, appropriate changes of therapy in a timely manner.

2.8 Professionalism/Affective Behavior

The student must fulfill the responsibilities for professional conduct as outlined on page 17 of the *Manual for Paramedic Students and Instructors*.

2.9 Communication

The student is responsible for establishing and maintaining effective communication with the patient and other personnel, and with all other persons during the patient contact, as needed.

2.10 Skill/IV Skill/ET Skill

This competency is used to document performance of skills. Some examples of skills are monitor application, use of an airway adjunct, defibrillation, medication administration, transcutaneous pacing, or spinal immobilization.

Performance of intravenous access (IV) and endotracheal intubation (ET) is also documented in this competency. IV and ET attempts are recorded as successful (first or second attempt) or as unsuccessful (first or second attempt).

2.10-A Cardiac Monitor Strip/Rhythm Interpretation

The student must secure a short (4 to 6 seconds in duration) monitor strip to this section of the Critique Form. The student must also identify the rhythm.

Section 3

3.1 Overall Score

The student receives a score (satisfactory/unsatisfactory) for his overall performance during the patient contact.

3.2 Instructor Comments

The instructor uses this part of the Critique Form to write additional comments regarding performance of a competency or skill. Comments should be objective and define why the performance of a competency was exceptional or unsatisfactory. The instructor can place the number of the competency in front of the written comments. For example:

> (2) Student failed to assess for obstructed airway (tongue) and did not place an oropharyngeal airway. Completion of initial assessment and placement of oral airway was accomplished by the instructor.

> The instructor should use this section to document an action plan. The action plan will consist of specific recommendations that are intended to improve the student's performance.

3.3 Student Comments

The student is *strongly encouraged* to complete this section. The student should use this space to respond to scores or comments entered on a Critique Form. For example:

> (2) I was holding the patient's airway open with a jaw thrust and had sent another student for an airway—if the instructor had not intervened I could have completed the initial assessment and treatment without his help.

> The student *must* document any significant difference of opinion (between the student and the instructor) prior to signing the form. Differences of opinion that are not supported by documentation in the student comments section will be viewed as unsupported allegations.

3.4 Signatures (Instructor and Student) and Date

The instructor must sign the Critique Form once all other sections of the form have been completed.

> The student must read and sign the Critique Form. The student's signature indicates only that the student has read the form. The signature does not indicate that the student agrees with the scores or instructor's comments. Once the student has signed the Critique Form, he should enter the date.

EMT-P Clinical Critique	Obs.	Rem.	TL	TLE

Circle each appropriate category: Pediatric   Geriatric   Trauma   Cardiac   Neuro   Respiratory   Gen. Med.   Psych.   OB

Section 1

Name: _____   Department: _____   Date: _____

Instructor: _____   Priority: 1   1-M   2   3

Pt. age _____   Pt. sex   M / F   CC : _____

Pt.'s Presentation, HPI, MOI:

Other students who witnessed this assessment:

Section 2   Score of: 1 = Unsatisfactory   2 = Unsatisfactory (parts satisfactory)   3 = Satisfactory

Instructors: *Circle both the word "Prompt" (and the skill that was prompted) to indicate that a prompt was given.*
Checkmarks will to indicate satisfactory skill performance.

Self-test: Student's actions: Safe?   Appropriate?   Timely?   Within Protocol?

Scene / Multi-   Assesses scene safety, need for additional personnel, and takes appropriate actions. Document ability
                            to delegate, multitask, and make decisions here.

1.   1   2   3   ++   (elapsed scene time:)

Prompt: Safety   # of Patients/Personnel   Task Delegation (specify)   Multitasking   Decisions (where to . . . , when to . . .)

Initial   Completes the initial assessment within thirty (30) seconds. Physically intervenes, within thirty (30)
                     seconds, to address, appropriately, problems found during the initial assessment.

2.   1   2   3   ++   (elapsed assessment time:)   (elapsed intervention time:)

Prompt: c-spine   Airway / Reposition / Adjunct   Breathing / O_2 / BVM   Circulation / Flat / CPR   Disability (AVPU)   Expose

---

History   Obtains chief complaint, pertinent history of present illness, and pertinent past medical history.

3.   1   2   3   ++   Associated Symptoms: CP   SOB   IDDM   H/A   N / V / D   (Recent) Trauma   Cough   Fever

Prompt: CC   HPI / PMH   PPTC   (O, P, Q, R, S, T, A, M, P, L, E)   Hospital Preference   Other:

Physical Exam   Completes all pertinent components of physical examination.

4.   1   2   3   ++   Stroke Scale   Blood Sugar   Rapid Trauma Assessment

Prompt: P   BP   RR   Lung Sounds   Pupils   Pulse Ox $EtCO_2$ PMS   Edema   Palpate   Rhythm   12 Lead

---

Protocols/Standard/Care   Intervenes within the framework of accepted medical standards, protocols, and standing orders.
                              Student must begin, or verablize, appropriate treatment regimen within three (3) minutes.

5.   1   2   3   ++   (elapsed time:)

Prompt: Differential Diagnosis   Knowledge of Protocols   Implementation

---

Revised 12-8-2004 by B. Nepon & B. Eberly

| **Reassess** | Reassesses, within five (5) minutes, for change in patient's condition or presentation. |

6. 1   2   3   ++   (elapsed time:)

Prompt: CC   Initial   Vital Signs   Lung Sounds   Blood Sugar   Pulse Ox   Pupils   PMS   Cardiac Rhythm   12 Lead

---

Change of Therapy   Changes, or verbalize change of, treatment, within thirty (30) seconds, following change in patient's condition or presentation.

7. 1   2   3   ++   (elapsed time:)

Prompt: Differential Diagnosis   Knowledge of Protocols   Implementation

---

Professional/Affective   Fulfills responsibilities for professional conduct and affective behavior as outlined in the *Manual for Paramedic Students and FTOs*.

8. 1   2   3   ++

Prompt: Honesty   Courtesy   Confidentiality   Accepts Responsibility   Accepts Constructive Criticism

---

Communication   Establishes and maintains effective lines of communication.

9. 1   2   3   ++   Establishes Communication   Maintains Communication

Prompt: Patient   Family   Witness   EMS Personnel   Other Personnel

---

Skill   Skill   Skill

10. 1   2   3   ++   1   2   3   ++   1   2   3   ++

IV / ET Skill   S1   S2   (elapsed time:)   Prompt:

1   2   3   ++   U1   U2

Cardiac Monitor Strip:

10-A. 1   2   3   ++

Rhythm Interpretation:

Prompt:

Section 3   Overall Score: Satisfactory   or   Unsatisfactory

(Instruction phase)   Were there... > 3 Prompts?   Have there been... > 3 Repetitive Prompts?

Instructor Comments: _____

_____

_____

Initial here if contact is "Unsatisfactory" based solely on severity of one prompt: _____   *Documentation is required.*

Student Comments:_____

_____

_____

_____

_____

Instructor Signature:_____   Student Signature: _____   Date: _____

Completion of Field Critique Form by Section

Section 1: Required Information

1.1 Student Name

1.2 Station Assignment

1.3 Date Patient Was Assessed

1.4 Instructor Name

1.5 County Incident Number

1.6 Medical or Trauma/Priority (Priority 1, 1-M, 2, or 3)

1.7 Patient Age and Sex

1.8 Chief Complaint/Reason for Activation of EMS System

1.9 Patient Presentation (include pertinent mechanism of injury and/or history of present illness)

Section 2: Scoring of Competency Indicators

- Score of 3 indicates satisfactory performance of a competency indicator.
  - ++ indicates exceptional performance (beyond entry level provider) of a competency indicator.
- Score of 2 indicates unsatisfactory performance of a competency indicator, although parts of the competency were performed satisfactorily.
- Score of 1 indicates unsatisfactory performance of a competency indicator.
- Each competency has space for an explanation of unsatisfactory performance. Students should refer to the instructor's comments to develop an action plan.

Elapsed Time: Certain competencies have space allotted for documentation of elapsed time. Failure to complete a skill or competency within the specified time frame may be cause for the student to receive an unsatisfactory score.

2.1 Scene/Multitask

Scene management includes scene safety, need for triage, and coordination of resources. The student will be required to delegate tasks. The student will be required to perform skills. Skill performance often must be accomplished simultaneously with task delegation and history-gathering. This skill is referred to as "multitasking."

2.2 Initial (Assessment and Treatment)

The student must complete the initial assessment and manage the patient appropriately. Refer to the Critique Form for time limits and interventions related to the initial assessment.

2.3 History

Includes patient's chief complaint (CC), history of present illness (HPI), and past medical history (PMH). The student must gather all pertinent information, relative to the patient's complaint or presentation.

2.4 Physical Exam

The student must complete a physical examination on each patient. This exam will include all pertinent exam procedures indicated by the patient's complaint or presentation. A list of prompt items for commonly used exam procedures is included in the Critique Form.

2.5 Protocols/Standard of Care

The patient must receive treatment that is in accordance with the local standard of care. The acceptable standard of care is outlined in the *State of Delaware Paramedic Standing Orders*.

2.6 Reassess

Change in the patient's condition may result from interventions or continuation of a disease, or injury, process. The student must reassess the patient for change in condition. Some changes in condition occur quickly. The student will be required to reassess in fewer than 5 minutes whenever there is a precipitous change in patient condition.

2.7 Change of Therapy

Change in the patient's condition may require change in therapy. The student must implement, or delegate, all appropriate changes of therapy in a timely manner.

2.8 Professionalism/Affective Behavior

The student must fulfill the responsibilities for professional conduct as outlined in this manual.

2.9 Communication

The student is responsible for establishing and maintaining effective communication with the patient and other personnel and with all other persons during the patient contact, as needed.

2.10 Skill/IV Skill/ET Skill

This competency is used to document performance of skills. Some examples of skills are monitor application, rhythm interpretation, using of an airway adjunct, defibrillation, medication administration, transcutaneous pacing, or spinal immobilization.

Performance of intravenous access (IV) and endotracheal intubation (ET) is also documented in this competency. IV and ET attempts are recorded as successful (first or second attempt) or as unsuccessful (first or second attempt).

2.11 Verbal Reports (Radio Report and Transfer of Care)

The student is required to contact medical control, give a concise and accurate report, and request orders as needed. This skill may be delegated, when appropriate. The student is also required to give a complete report and transfer patient care to the appropriate staff member of the receiving medical facility.

2.12 Written Report

The student is required to provide complete documentation of patient assessment and treatment on a Delaware Paramedic Care Report form. Reports should include all pertinent patient information, as well as information required for quality improvement data fields.

Section 3

3.1 Overall Score

The student receives a grade (satisfactory/unsatisfactory) for his overall performance during the patient contact.

3.2 Instructor Comments

The instructor uses this part of the Critique Form to write additional comments regarding performance of a competency or skill. Comments should be objective and must define why the performance of a competency was exceptional or unsatisfactory. The instructor can place the number of the competency in front of the written comments. For example:

(2) Student failed to assess for obstructed airway (tongue) and did not place an oropharyngeal airway. Completion of initial assessment and placement of oral airway was accomplished by instructor.

The instructor should use this section to document an action plan. The action plan will consist of specific recommendations that are intended to improve the student's performance.

3.3 Student Comments

The student is *strongly encouraged* to complete this section. The student should use this space to respond to scores or comments entered on a Critique Form. For example:

> (2) I was holding the patient's airway open with a jaw thrust and had sent BLS for an airway—if the instructor had not intervened I could have completed the initial assessment and treatment without her help.

The student *must* document any significant difference of opinion (between the student and the instructor) prior to signing the form. Differences of opinion that are not supported by documentation in the student comments section will be viewed as unsupported allegations.

3.4 Signatures (Instructor and Student) and Date

The instructor must sign the Critique Form once all other sections of the form have been completed.

The student must read and sign the Critique Form. The student's signature indicates only that the student has read the form. The signature does not mean that the student agrees with the scores or instructor's comments. Once the student has signed the Critique Form, he should enter the date.

EMT-P Field Critique	Obs.	Rem.	TM	TL	TLE

Circle each appropriate category: Pediatric Geriatric Trauma Cardiac Neuro Respiratory Gen. Med. Psych. OB

Section 1

Name:	Station:	Date:

Instructor:	Run #:	Priority: 1 1-M 2 3

Pt. age / sex:	CC :

Pt.'s Presentation, HPI, MOI:

Section 2   Score of: 1 = Unsatisfactory   2 = Unsatisfactory (parts satisfactory)   3 = Satisfactory

FTOs: *Circle both the word "Prompt" (and the skill that was prompted) to indicate that a prompt was given.*
Checkmark will indicate satisfactory skill performance.

Self-Test: Student's actions: Timely?   Appropriate?   Safe?   Within Protocol?

Scene / Multi-   Assesses scene safety, need for additional personnel, and takes appropriate actions. Document ability
to delegate, multitask, and make decisions here.

1. 1   2   3   ++   (elapsed scene time:)

Prompt: Safety   # of Patients/Personnel   Task Delegation (specify)   Multitasking   Decisions (where to . . . , when to . . .)

Initial   Completes the initial assessment within thirty (30) seconds. Physically intervenes, within thirty (30)
seconds, to address problems found during the initial assessment.

2. 1   2   3   ++   (elapsed assessment time:)   (elapsed intervention time:)

Prompt: c-spine   Airway / Reposition / Adjunct   Breathing / O_2 / BVM   Circulation / Flat / CPR   Disability (AVPU)   Expose

---

History   Obtains chief complaint, pertinent history of present illness, and pertinent past medical history.

3. 1   2   3   ++   Associated Symptoms: CP   SOB   IDDM   H/A   N / V / D   Recent: Trauma   Cough   Fever

Prompt: CC   HPI / PMH   Initial   (O, P, Q, R, S, T, A, M, P, L, E)   Hospital Preference   Other:

Physical Exam   Completes all pertinent components of physical examination.

4. 1   2   3   ++   Stroke Scale   Blood Sugar   Rapid Trauma Assessment

Prompt: P   BP   RR   Lung Sounds   Pupils   Pulse Ox $EtCO_2$ PMS   Edema   Palpate   Rhythm 12 Lead

---

Protocols/Standard/Care   Intervenes within the framework of accepted medical standards, protocols, and standing orders.
Student must begin appropriate treatment regimen within three (3) minutes.

5. 1   2   3   ++   (elapsed time:)

Prompt: Differential Diagnosis   Knowledge of Protocols   Implementation

Revised 12-18-2005 by B. Nepon and B. Eberly

Reassess	Reassesses, within five (5) minutes, for change in patient's condition or presentation.

6. 1   2   3   ++   (elapsed time:)

Prompt: CC   Initial   Vital Signs   Breath   Sounds   Pulse Ox   Pupils   PMS

Change of Therapy   Changes course of treatment, within thirty (30) seconds, following change in patient's condition or presentation.

7. 1   2   3   ++   (elapsed time:)

Prompt: Differential Diagnosis   Knowledge of Protocols   Implementation

---

Professional/Affective   Fulfills responsibilities for professional conduct and affective behavior as outlined in the *Manual for Paramedic Students and FTOs*.

8. 1   2   3   ++

Prompt: Honesty   Courtesy   Confidentiality   Accepts Responsibility   Accepts Constructive Criticism

---

Communication   Establishes and maintains effective lines of communication.

9. 1   2   3   ++   Establishes Communication   Maintains Communication

Prompt: Patient   Family   Witness   EMS Personnel   Other Personnel

---

   Skill   Skill   Skill

10. 1   2   3   ++   1   2   3   ++   1   2   3   ++

   IV / ET Skill   S1   S2   (elapsed time:)   Prompt:

   1   2   3   ++   U1   U2

   Verbal Reports   (Radio)   Contacts medical control. Gives concise report and requests orders (PRN).

                             (Transfer)   Gives complete report to appropriate staff member of receiving facility.

11. 1   2   3   ++

Prompt:

   Written Report   Provides complete documentation on Delaware patient care report form.

12. 1   2   3   ++

Prompt:

Section 3   **Overall Score:**   Satisfactory   ++   or   Unsatisfactory

(Instruction phase)   Were there... > 3 Prompts?   Have there been... > 3 Repetitive Prompts?

Instructor Comments: _____

_____

_____

Initial here if contact is "Unsatisfactory" based solely on severity of one prompt: _____ *Documentation is required.*

Student / Candidate Comments: _____

_____

_____

_____

Instructor Signature:_____ Student Signature: _____ Date: _____

Assigned Tasks (Field Internship Only)

As a student enrolled in the Paramedic Technology Program you have the responsibility to:

- Arrive at the designated work site at least 15 minutes prior to the normal shift change. The instructor should document time of arrival.
- Initiate equipment and vehicle inspections. This duty may be relieved, or temporarily suspended, by the instructor.
- Complete assigned documentation in a time-appropriate manner. Such documentation would include:
  - Vehicle checklists
  - Medical equipment checklists
  - Patient care report forms
  - (EMS agency) run log forms
- Assist in restocking of medical supplies and equipment unless otherwise assigned.
- Assist in cleaning and maintenance of the vehicle and medical equipment. Duty to perform other school-related tasks may be cause for the student to be excused from cleaning and maintenance duties.
- Not end their assigned shift without permission from their instructor.
- Complete study assignment given by the instructor to improve or enhance competency performance.
- Initiate activities to effectively use "down time."

Professional Conduct and Affective Behavior

As a student enrolled in the Paramedic Technology Program you have the responsibility to:

- Speak and act in a calm manner. The instructor must document inappropriate behavior. This behavior may be documented on any of these forms: Clinical Critique, Field Critique, Daily Clinical Tally, or Instructor Checklist.
- Assist the student who is in the role of team leader.
- Avoid conflict with other healthcare and emergency service personnel. If a student's disagreement is related to patient care, the student must make every effort to resolve the disagreement in an unobtrusive manner. Public disagreements slow delivery of care and are unprofessional. Ultimately, the highest medical authority (usually FTO or instructor) is responsible for patient care and therefore must be deferred to by the student.
- Treat the patient with respect, including the preservation of patient confidentiality.
- Establish and maintain effective lines of verbal and nonverbal communications.
- Be honest and courteous when interacting with: patient, family members, bystanders, and other emergency service providers.
- Be receptive to constructive feedback. Occasionally, a student will have a difference of opinion (with the instructor) that has not been resolved to his satisfaction. The student should document the issue, or problem, and contact the program coordinator.
- Accept responsibility for your actions. The student should not make excuses to explain why he did something incorrectly or why he failed to accomplish a skill that needed to be performed. It is in the student's best interest to accept responsibility. Time is more wisely invested developing a plan of corrective action rather than being used to make excuses.

- Adhere to the policies and procedures of the organization where they are participating in the clinical or field experience. This includes the organization's policy on smoking.
- Maintain a professional appearance by adhering to the following criteria:
  - Wear the uniform assigned for the specific patient care area.
  - Long hair must be positioned above shoulder level.
  - Watches and wedding bands are the *only* acceptable jewelry for men.
  - Watches, wedding bands, and one pair of small stud earrings (earlobe) are the *only* acceptable jewelry for women.
  - All potentially offensive tattoos must be covered.
  - Clear fingernail polish is the *only* acceptable nail polish color.
  - Fingernails must be trimmed (not greater than 1/8" past the end of the finger).
  - Identification badges are required at all times (when a student is at a clinical or field clinical site).
  - Additional appearance criteria may apply to students who are also employee's of municipal EMS organizations.

Elapsed Time Guidelines

- Patient care must be accomplished in a timely manner. The instructor is ultimately responsible for care of the patient and must ensure that assessments and therapies are completed within reasonable time frames.
- The instructor must document elapsed time for the following skills and for scene times. Examples of maximum allowable elapsed times are:
  - Initial Assessment: 30 seconds (from time of initial patient contact by student to completion of verbal report)
  - Initial Interventions: 30 seconds (from time a deficit is detected until the student physically intervenes; exception is a 15-second limit for manual reposition of the airway)
  - Protocols/Standard Care: 3 minutes (from time of initial patient contact until student begins appropriate treatment regimen)
  - Reassess: 5 minutes (from time of initial patient assessment)
  - Change of Therapy: 30 seconds (from recognition of change until student begins appropriate therapy)
  - (IV) Skill: 5 minutes (clinical) 3 minutes (field) (from application of tourniquet until line is secured and flow rate adjusted; IV setup may be delegated)
  - (ET) Skill: 1 minute (from placement of the laryngoscope blade to verification of placement; verification includes EDD, check for breath sounds, check for epigastric sounds, and capnography as indicated by protocol)
  - **On-Scene Time (medical) (from time of arrival to departure): 15 minutes
  - **On-Scene Time (trauma) (from time of arrival to departure): 10 minutes
- It is both the right and the responsibility of the instructor to modify elapsed time requirements in the presence of mitigating factors. If the instructor deviates from the written *Elapsed Time Guidelines*, he should provide a clear justification of that decision. The student is not held accountable for time limits that are more stringent than those described above.

The Daily Log Form will be printed on the outside of the envelope that contains the student's Critique Forms. The student will place the accrued documentation (Critique Forms, patient care reports, and the Instructor Checklist) into the envelope. The instructor will then complete and sign the Daily Log form.

Daily Log Form

Date: _____   **Unit:** _____

Instructor: _____   **Student:** _____

Pt.	Incident #	Patient: Age, Sex, Complaint	TM/TL/TLE	Feedback
1				Y/N
2				Y/N
3				Y/N
4				Y/N
5				Y/N

Initials: Instructor: _____   Student: _____

Instructor Checklist

Instructor: _____   **Station:** _____

Student: _____   **Time of arrival:** _____

1. Attire and Equipment   Satisfactory ____ Unsatisfactory ____
2. Equipment Checks   Satisfactory ____ Unsatisfactory ____ N/A ____
3. Documentation (logs)   Satisfactory ____ Unsatisfactory ____ N/A ____
4. Restocking   Satisfactory ____ Unsatisfactory ____ N/A ____
5. Cleaning/Maintenance   Satisfactory ____ Unsatisfactory ____ N/A ____
6. Completes self-study assignments Satisfactory ____ Unsatisfactory ____ N/A ____
7. Effectively uses down time   Satisfactory ____ Unsatisfactory ____ N/A ____
8. Relieved for end of shift   Satisfactory ____ Unsatisfactory ____
9. Affect/Professional Conduct   Satisfactory ____ Unsatisfactory ____

Instructor Comments:

_____
_____
_____

Student Comments:

_____
_____
_____

Signatures:

Instructor: _____   Date: _____

Student: _____   Date: _____

PART 2: For Students and Instructors

General Criteria

The student may have a question or comment about the material found in this manual. These questions and comments should be submitted, in writing, to the program coordinator. The program coordinator will respond within five business days.

Students should use any comments documented on their Clinical Critique Forms or Field Critique Forms as recommendations for an action plan. An action plan is a directed, or self-directed, thought process used to improve or correct performance.

Each course (i.e., clinical internship semester, field internship semester) is divided into three phases: observation, instruction, and evaluation. Each semester is potentially two weeks longer than the total time allotted for the three phases. The extra two weeks may be used to provide additional education for those students who are meeting criteria for successful completion or to provide remediation for students who are not meeting criteria for successful completion. Remediation may be offered in either the instruction or evaluation phases.

Verbalization

The student is responsible for verbalizing activities during the patient contact to the instructor. For example, immediately following completion of chief complaint and initial assessment the student might tell the instructor "the airway is patent, breathing is fast and shallow with equal chest rise; I want to apply oxygen 15 L/min by nonre-breather; the pulse is fast, regular, and strong, the skin is pale in color, warm and dry and the patient is alert and oriented, and the complaint is chest pain." The student's verbalization of the initial assessment and appropriate therapy (oxygen) serve to inform the instructor that the student completed the assessment and initiated appropriate initial interventions.

The instructor may acknowledge (verbally or physically) that he has heard questions and answers related to chief complaint, history of present illness, and past medical history. Whenever an instructor gives these cues, the student will not be expected to repeat this information to the instructor.

The instructor will generally see the student perform physical exams and skills. The student is, however, responsible for reporting the results of the exams and skills. For example:

- Lung sounds: "Clear except for crackles in both bases."
- Blood pressure: "122 over 78."
- Medication administration: "I'm giving two aspirin—total of 162 mg PO."
- Monitor: "It's sinus tach on the rhythm strip, with ST depression."
- Chest/breathing: "Equal chest rise, accessory muscle use and retractions."

The instructor is responsible for observing, prompting, and documenting student performance (e.g., histories, exams, skills). However, the responsibilities of patient care occasionally make it impossible for the instructor to witness all components of a student's performance. The student's verbalization ensures that the instructor does not miss parts of the student's performance.

The instructor may be distracted and not witness performance of a skill. Students might not receive a satisfactory grade if they have not verbalized the procedure and the result.

Occasionally, the instructor will ask the student to explain the thought processes that caused him to pursue a certain course of action. This is done to ensure that the instructor understands the decision-making process used by the student.

Prompts

Prompts are an integral part of the instruction and evaluation process. An instructor will use prompts to improve student performance (e.g., scene management, medical history questions, exam procedures, treatment regimens or skill performance). Prompts benefit the patient by ensuring that care is not delayed. Prompts are designed to help the student perform skills properly and to perform those skills at the most appropriate time within the assessment and treatment sequence.

Prompts made by the instructor will be documented on the Critique Form. The program coordinator will use this data (numbers and types of prompts) to look for trends in performance.

Example: The student (first week/instruction phase/clinical internship) accurately reports that the airway is compromised by the tongue ("has fast and shallow snoring respirations") but does not undertake manual control of the jaw or call for an airway adjunct. The instructor asks the student if he can do anything to help the patient. The student performs a jaw thrust, calls for a nasal airway adjunct and oxygen at 15 L/m via nonrebreather, and completes the initial exam. In this situation, the patient receives care that is timely and appropriate and the student receives a satisfactory grade for the *initial* competency.

Although a competency, or skill, *may* be graded satisfactory (with prompt) the instructor has discretion in the grading process. A student who requires more than three prompts will generally receive an unsatisfactory evaluation. A student who receives more than three similar (repetitive) prompts for the same skill on successive patient contacts will generally receive an unsatisfactory evaluation.

Example: The student has noted shortness of breath (chief complaint tachypnea, bradypnea, accessory muscle use, retractions, etc.) during the initial assessment for five patients in a two-week period. The instructors have documented that prompts were required for application of oxygen therapy on each of these patients. The student is in the instruction phase of the clinical internship and the instructors each scored the *initial/primary* competency as "satisfactory with prompt for oxygen therapy." The program coordinator will review the Clinical Critique forms, note the recurring problem, change the scoring to unsatisfactory for the last two patients, advise the student of the scoring change, assist the student with additional action plan strategies, and advise all instructors that this student has demonstrated a recurring deficiency. Further, the program coordinator, with involvement from the program medical director, may adjust scoring.

Performance of a competency, or skill, that is successfully completed with the aid of a prompt may be scored unsatisfactory, at the discretion of the instructor. The student will receive an unsatisfactory score whenever prompts are given for a critical (shaded) competency during the evaluation phase(s). The only exception is when the student's assessment and treatment regimen are within acceptable parameters (see Elapsed Time). However, the instructor prompts for faster skill performance to provide more expeditious care to an unstable patient.

Documentation

The student is responsible for documenting on the Critique Form any unresolved difference of opinion between the student and the instructor.

Remediation

Remediation (for the purposes of this educational program) means instruction designed to correct unsatisfactory performance of one or more specific skills. Instructors routinely remediate paramedic students. The instructor is required to give every student immediate verbal feedback for every patient contact. The instructor also is required to document this feedback on the Critique Form. These processes provide a built-in remediation for this program's process of instruction and evaluation.

The primary goal of remediation is to give the student a mechanism to improve his performance. A student will receive remedial instruction (remediation) whenever a competency is not performed correctly. The following are a few generic examples of unsatisfactory performance that would be cause for remediation:

- Competency performance is incorrect (e.g., facemask of bag-mask device applied upside down).
- Competency performance exceeded allowable time parameters.
- Student had difficulty managing multiple tasks simultaneously.
- Student exhibited unacceptable affective behavior.
- Sequencing of assessment and treatment skills, or competencies, is unacceptable.
- Treatment regimen was not appropriate.

Remediation provided to a student during either the clinical or field semesters will routinely incorporate *at least* three of the following types of remedial interaction:

- Verbal prompts (given to a student)
- Physical prompts (given to a student)
- Documentation of prompts (given to a student)
- Verbal feedback (given to a student, following a patient contact)
- Written recommendations for performance improvement (given to a student)
- Placement (of a student) into a specific period of remediation

For example, continuing from the earlier example, the student receives (1) a verbal prompt for applying oxygen, (2) verbal feedback about the reason for this prompt (following the patient contact), and (3) documentation on a Critique Form that this prompt occurred.

Verbal Prompts

Instructors will use verbal prompts such as "oxygen," "past history," "lung sounds," or "what protocol are you going to follow?" in an effort to induce satisfactory performance.

Physical Prompts

Instructors will use physical prompts in an effort to induce satisfactory performance. An example of such a prompt would be when an instructor uses a prearranged signal (cupped hand over instructor's face) to prompt the student to give the patient oxygen via nonrebreather mask.

Documentation of Prompts

Instructors are required to document any prompts (verbal, physical, or inadvertent) that occur during a patient contact. The student will review this documentation when reviewing the Critique Form from that patient contact. The student should use this documentation to develop an action plan. The program coordinator will use accumulated documentation (an accumulation of Critique Forms from multiple patient contacts) to determine if there is a developing pattern of unsatisfactory performance. When a pattern (of similar prompts) is detected, the program coordinator will assist the student in developing a formal plan for remediation.

Verbal Feedback

Instructors will give the student verbal feedback as soon as possible following a patient contact. This feedback is not intended to be comprehensive in nature. Verbal feedback is intended to address portions of the preceding patient contact that require immediate attention. Patient contacts frequently occur with little time between incidents. On those occasions that contacts occur in rapid succession, the instructor will be unable to complete a written Critique Form before the next contact is under way. Verbal feedback ensures that the student has enough information to adjust his performance on the subsequent patient contact. The goal is to eliminate repeated mistakes. The instructor must clearly inform the student that a patient contact is satisfactory or unsatisfactory prior to the end of the shift.

Written Recommendations (Action Plan)

Instructors should make recommendations for performance improvement in the Instructor's Comments section of the Critique Form. The program coordinator makes recommendations for improvement after a review of multiple Critique Forms indicates a pattern of performance that requires extensive remediation. These recommendations are generally included in periodic written evaluations that will be given to the students.

Placement into Remediation Phase

If the student is unable to demonstrate satisfactory performance following the culmination of verbal prompts, physical prompts, documentation (Critique Forms), verbal feedback, and written recommendations, the program coordinator will place the student into a formal remediation phase.

The student will be removed from the instruction/evaluation phase and placed in a remediation phase. Remediation will generally be provided by faculty personnel from Delaware Technical and Community College. This phase will not exceed two weeks in length. Once remediation is completed, the student will be moved back into either the instruction phase or the evaluation phase. Continued unsatisfactory performance, following remediation, may result in dismissal from the program. Semesters (clinical and field) are limited to a finite amount of time. Delaware Technical and Community College establishes the time limits for each semester. If a student is unable to successfully complete a semester, as a result of time lost to remediation, that student will receive a failing grade.

Occasionally, a student receives large numbers, *and* a large variety, of prompts. This student will not be eligible for a formal process of remediation. The formal process for remediation is designed to address deficiencies in one, or two, specific skills.

Criteria for Successful Completion of Clinical Internship

Instruction Phase (Observation 1 Week, Instruction 5 Weeks)

The instruction phase of the student's clinical internship is composed of two parts. One part of the clinical instruction is a variety of *specialty rotations* (i.e., anesthesia, obstetrics, pediatrics, paramedic unit). Students are expected to observe procedures, perform certain assigned skills, and conduct themselves in a professional manner during these rotations. Daily Clinical Tally Sheets (forms) will be used to document the student's performance for all patient contacts. The student will not receive grades for any of the specialty rotations. The assigned preceptor (nurse, FTO, physician) will use one form to record a summary of observed procedures (number and type of skills) performed and affective behavior for each day of specialty rotation. Students will be assigned to specialty rotations throughout the course of their clinical internship.

The remaining part of the clinical instruction phase takes place in the emergency department of hospitals that have clinical agreements with the college. These emergency departments provide a learning environment for paramedic students. Paramedic instructors will teach and evaluate students in these emergency departments. Paramedic students will be instructed, remediated, and evaluated on all competencies listed on the Clinical Critique Form. When an instructor is not available, students may be assigned to a nurse preceptor who will assign skills and document skill performance on a Daily Clinical Tally Sheet.

In the emergency department portion of the clinical internship, a Clinical Critique Form will be completed and a score assigned for each patient contact that is monitored by a paramedic instructor.

During both the clinical instruction and clinical evaluation phases, the student may receive prompts that are designed to improve assessment and treatment skills. These prompts are also designed to help students develop a rhythm in the clinical environment and to expedite delivery of patient care. All prompts should be documented on the Clinical Critique Form. While the student is in the clinical instruction phase, competencies that require prompts may be scored (satisfactory or unsatisfactory) according to the number of prompts on a single patient contact and/or according to the number of similar prompts the student has previously received. A student who has received more than three repetitive prompts (prompts that are repeated on different patient contacts) will be given an *unsatisfactory* score. A student who has received more than three separate prompts (on one patient contact) will be given an *unsatisfactory* score.

Unsolicited or inadvertent prompts by persons other than the instructor will occur. Scoring may be impacted by these prompts. The instructor will consider the impact of these prompts before scoring the patient contact.

In order to complete the instruction phase of the clinical semester each student must manage:

- At least 10 patient contacts (Priorities 1, 2, and 3 combined) with at least a 50% success rate
- At least 8 patient contacts (Priority 2 or greater) with at least a 50% success rate
- At least 1 Priority 1-M patient contact (satisfactory, or unsatisfactory)

Any (documented) skill performance that occurs during this phase will count toward the number of skills that are required to successfully complete the clinical semester.

The student must also achieve a consistent level of performance to successfully complete this phase of the clinical internship. Whenever a student requires prompting to complete a patient contact, the nature of the prompt is documented on the appropriate critique form. The program coordinator monitors the number and types of prompts throughout the semester. A student who requires an excessive number of prompts will not be able to achieve a consistent level of performance.

Evaluation Phase (5 weeks)

Following successful completion of the clinical instruction phase, the student will then move to the clinical evaluation phase of the clinical internship.

In this phase a Clinical Critique Form will be completed for each patient contact. A grade will be assigned to each form. Every time a student is prompted more than once (for critical competencies only), the student will receive an unsatisfactory score. A student who has received more than three repetitive prompts (prompts that are repeated on different patient contacts) will be given an *unsatisfactory* score.

In order to successfully complete the clinical semester, the student must, in the evaluation phase, manage:

- At least 12 patient contacts (Priorities 1, 2 and 3 combined) with at least a 75% success rate
- At least 8 patient contacts (Priority 2 or greater) with at least a 75% success rate
- At least 1 satisfactory Priority 1-M patient contact

Criteria for Successful Completion of Field Internship

Criteria for Completion of Field Internship (Instruction Phase)

The instruction phase of the field internship is composed of two parts. The first part is the 1-week period during which the instructor serves as a template for the students. The instructor serves as the team leader during this period. In that role, the instructor demonstrates to the students how they are to perform in the field (out-of-hospital environment). The instructor may also choose to allow the students to alternate as team leader and team member.

The instructor will provide a large amount of instruction and direction during the observation portion of the instruction phase. The purpose of this period is to demonstrate to the students the roles and responsibilities they will assume as team leaders and team members. This observation period allows the student to see the parameters within which he must perform in order to be successful in the field instruction phase.

The second part of the field instruction phase is the (approximately) 5-week period during which the instructor will no longer assume the role of team leader. The students will alternate in the team leader and team member roles whenever there are two students on a unit. During this period the instructor will still provide direction in the form of feedback and prompting. When necessary, the instructor will prompt the student to improve skill performance.

During this (approximately) 5-week period, a Critique Form will be completed on each patient contact. A satisfactory or unsatisfactory grade will be assigned to each form. A student may still achieve a satisfactory grade even if a prompt was received during the course of patient contact. The instructor, however, always has the authority to score any prompted skill performance as unsatisfactory.

During both the field instruction and field evaluation phases the student will receive prompts that are designed to improve assessment and treatment skills. These prompts are also designed to help students develop a rhythm in the field environment and to expedite delivery of patient care. All prompts must be documented on the appropriate Critique Form. While the student is in the instruction phase, competencies that require prompts may be scored (as satisfactory or unsatisfactory) according to the number of prompts on a single patient contact. Scoring may be affected by the number of repetitive prompts which the student has received. More than three repetitive prompts (repeated prompts for a certain skill, occurring on different patient contacts) will be cause for an unsatisfactory score. Documentation of more than three separate prompts on one patient contact will also be cause for an unsatisfactory score.

Inadvertent (unsolicited) prompts by persons other than the instructor will occur. Scoring may be impacted by these prompts. The instructor will consider the impact of these prompts before scoring the patient contact.

In order to successfully complete this portion of the field instruction phase a student must manage:

- At least 25 patient contacts (priorities 1, 2, 3, combined) with at least a 60% success rate

- At least 20 patient contacts, Priority 2 or greater with at least a 60% success rate
- At least 1 satisfactory Priority 1-M patient
- A skill success rate (IV, and other skills) of at least 50% (all skills are per attempt, not per patient)

Criteria for Completion of Field Internship (Evaluation Phase)

Following successful completion of the instruction phase, each student will move to the evaluation phase of the field internship. Ideally, the instructor will serve primarily as an evaluator of each student's performance. There will be little intervention by the instructor unless the instructor must intervene to ensure that the patient receives timely and appropriate care. Students will alternate in the team leader and team member roles whenever there are two students on a unit. A prompt given during the evaluation phase *may* result in an unsatisfactory score if the prompt was to correct an error that was critical to patient care. Generally, whenever a student is prompted more than one time (for critical competencies only) he will receive an unsatisfactory overall score.

In order to successfully complete the evaluation phase, a student must manage:
- At least 25 patient contacts (Priorities 1, 2, 3, combined) with at least a 75% success rate
- At least 20 patient contacts, Priority 2 or greater, with at least a 75% success rate
- At least 5 patient contacts, Priority 1 or greater (1-M), with at least a 60% success rate
- At least 1 satisfactory priority 1-M patient contact
- A skill success rate of at least 50% for IVs, and 75% for all other skills (per attempt)

Failure to properly complete the initial assessment and initial interventions on any Priority 1 patient may result in a case review by the Program Medical Director. Following the case review, the medical director may recommend that the student be dismissed from the program.

During this phase the student must successfully manage at least two patients from each of the following patient categories: respiratory, trauma, cardiac, altered mental status, and geriatric. A patient may qualify for more than one category.

A student may be extended in any of the three phases of the field internship. Extensions can only be arranged by, and at the discretion of, the program coordinator.

Priority 1-M

Successful completion of either clinical or field semesters requires that each student manage a predetermined number of Priority 1-M patients. Successful management of these complex situations provides the most definitive measure of the student's ability to provide acceptable patient care to unstable patients. Typically, management of Priority 1-M patients involves short scene times, rapid decision making, rapid accomplishment of skills, and decisive use of personnel.

Encounters with Priority 1-M patients are infrequent. Some examples of typical Priority 1-M patients are:
- CHF requiring CPAP, medications (albuterol, NTG, vasopressors), or volume fluids
- Multi-system trauma with significant hypotension and/or GCS less than 11
- Trauma patients requiring DFI, or needle decompression, with an $EtCO_2$ >15 mm Hg
- Cardiac arrest patients with return of spontaneous circulation (ROSC)
- ACS patients requiring electrical intervention (pacing, cardioversion)
- ACS patients requiring additional treatment for hypotension or respiratory compromise
- Respiratory compromise requiring endotracheal intubation
- Cardiac arrest with multiple rhythm changes

Responsibility for Classification

FTOs are very busy during the field internship semester. FTOs will not be required to make a decision about whether a patient contact meets the criteria for a Priority 1-M. Although an FTO has the option to classify a contact as a 1-M, the field internship coordinator will review all patient contacts. The coordinator will assign the most appropriate priority.

Occasionally, a student will not have the opportunity to manage a significant amount of 1-M patients. The program coordinator, and the medical director, may elect to waive the requirements for Priority 1-M patients. This would most likely occur when a student has managed more than five Priority 1 patients but has had a limited opportunity to manage 1-M patients.

Minimum Skills Requirements

In order to complete the Paramedic Technology Program, the student must have documentation of successful skill performance for the minimum number (shown below) of the following skills:

Skill	Required in Clinical	Required in Field	Minimum Required
IV (minimum success rate 60%)	8	1	10
Pediatric vital signs	5	0	10
PO medication administration	2	0	5
IM medication administration	2	0	2
IV push medication administration	5	5	10
SQ medication administration	2	0	2
Transdermal medication administration	1	0	2
SL medication administration	2	0	6
12-lead interpretation	5	0	10
Nebulized medication administration	2	0	5
Complete vital signs (HR/RR/BP)	15	15	30
Dynamic rhythm interpretation	10	10	20
Adventitious lung sounds	10	0	10
CPR (chest compressions)	1	0	1
Application of oxygen	10	0	10
Bag-mask ventilation	2	0	2
Airway clearance (suction)	2	0	5
Pupil check	5	0	10
Application of pulse oximetry	5	0	10
Blood glucometry	2	0	5
Orotracheal intubations	5	0	5

Routing of Paperwork

During the field internship semester, four types of documents are generated every shift:

1. The instructor generates a Field Critique Form for each patient contact, whenever the student is in a TL or TLE role.
2. The instructor generates a Daily Log form (every day) to document the number and type of patient contacts.
3. The instructor generates a Daily Checklist to document student behaviors that occur outside of patient contacts.
4. The student completes a Questionnaire each day. This is an important tool for evaluating the performance of the instructors.

An *EDIN Report* is generated for each patient contact and is to be attached to the coinciding Field Critique.

These items will be secured within an envelope at the end of each day. The instructor will then sign the Daily Log Form. It is the responsibility of the student to collect all paperwork at the end of each shift. It is also the responsibility of the student to deliver paperwork to the field internship coordinator at the beginning of each biweekly lab.

Grievance Procedure

The field internship semester is designed to provide a structured environment. The intent is to afford the student an opportunity to successfully complete the field internship. A situation may occur, however, that disrupts the student's progress. Examples of such situations include, but are not limited to:

- (Perceived) personality clash with an instructor
- (Perceived) harassment by the instructor or other EMS provider personnel
- (Perceived) physical threat to the student
- (Perceived) lack of confidentiality on the part of the instructor
- (Perceived) scheduling that is deemed, by the student, to be unfair

If the student has been exposed to such a situation, he should first attempt to resolve the conflict through discussion with his instructor. Both the student and the instructor should document the nature of the conflict. They should also document any efforts made to resolve the problem. The field internship coordinator should then be contacted within 24 hours. If the field internship coordinator is not available, the program coordinator should be contacted.

If the student has been unsuccessful in resolving the issue, or if he does not believe he can safely attempt resolution, the field internship coordinator should be contacted immediately. If the field internship coordinator is not available, the program coordinator should be contacted.

The student may believe the issue has not been adequately addressed (by representatives of the Paramedic Technology Program). In such an instance, he should consult the *Student Handbook*. Other resources are available at the college, outside of the Paramedic Technology Program, to assist the student.

Similarly, if the student believes that an action taken by the field internship coordinator is unacceptable, the program coordinator should be contacted. If there is no satisfactory resolution, the student should consult the *Student Handbook* and utilize other available resources.

Requirements for Program Completion

- Complete all program coursework with a "C" or better.
- Consistently demonstrate behaviors consistent with the profession.
- Obtain and maintain certification as a National Registry Emergency Medical Technician-Basic (prerequisite for internship as paramedic student).
- Participate in an oral board consisting minimally of the Program Director and Medical Director.

Receipt Page (for Students)

The guidelines included in this *Manual for Paramedic Students and Instructors* were developed, in part, to benefit students. This manual should be retained throughout the course of the student's field evaluation process. It should serve as a reference guide for the paramedic student.

To: _____

           First   Middle initial   Last

                       (paramedic student)

Please print your name, sign your name, and write date of signature in the designated places. This page will be retained as verification that you have received a copy of the *Manual for Paramedic Students and Instructors*.

                                                Date: _____

_____

      (signature of paramedic student)

Witness: _____

                (signature)

Title: _____   Date: _____

        (job title of witness)

PART 3: For Instructors

Purpose, Goal, and Objectives

Purpose

The purpose of this section of the *Manual* is to establish guidelines that should be used when paramedic instructors are teaching and evaluating students. The guidelines in Section 3 are to be used in conjunction with those found in Sections 1 and 2 of this manual.

Goal

Use of the guidelines found in the *Manual* will promote thorough, but equitable, instruction and evaluation of paramedic students. The goal is to establish performance expectations that present a comprehensive educational opportunity to every paramedic student. This goal must be accomplished without compromising standards of patient care. Most of those standards are defined in the *State of Delaware Paramedic Standing Orders*.

Objectives

Instructors should use the information contained in this manual to help them:
- Understand the general operational guidelines for paramedic instructors.
- Understand the terminology that is unique to this process of instruction and evaluation.
- Understand the criteria for satisfactory performance of skills and competencies.
- Understand the techniques used to document skill performance.
- Understand the criteria for satisfactory management of a patient contact.

The instructor acknowledges receipt of this manual by signing the receipt page of this document. Once the instructor has signed and dated the receipt page, he should remove this page from the manual. This page should then be delivered to the program coordinator.

Guidelines for Instructors

As an instructor for the Paramedic Technology Program, you are responsible to:
- Be familiar with the *Manual for Paramedic Students and Instructors*.
- Apply the guidelines set forth in the *Manual* when teaching and evaluating paramedic students. The instructor should pay particular attention to Section 2 of the *Manual*. Section 2 reiterates techniques used to teach and evaluate paramedic students. The instructors should recognize the guidelines and techniques included in Section 2. Each instructor has been exposed to this material in FTO workshops, and in FTO continuing education classes. The material is included in this manual, in part, as a reminder to the instructor. The instructor should prompt the student whenever the student's skill performance is at risk of being: incomplete, incorrect, or too slow. The instructor's first responsibility is to make sure that all patients receive care that is timely and appropriate. By using "prompts" the instructor gives the student the opportunity to perform all pertinent skills in a time-appropriate manner.
  - Complete all required documentation. Refer to Parts 1 and 2 of this manual.

- Teach students. There will be occasions when a student is not involved in patient care, or in other duties related to the clinical or field internships. In such an instance, the instructor should make himself available to review material related to the student's course of studies.
- Identify the student's areas of weakness. Whenever feasible, the instructor should devise a plan of self-study that the student can use to address these weaknesses. When time permits, the instructor may suggest that the student utilize "downtime" to conduct this regimen of self-study.
- Ensure that each patient receives care consistent with the various standards that apply to paramedics working within the Delaware EMS system. Whenever a student fails to provide appropriate care the instructor must assume the role of team leader.

- Not release information, regarding patients or students, to any person or agency that is not directly involved in the paramedic technology program.
- Not substitute his own personal "standard of care" when use of an approved (Standing Orders) protocol is appropriate to the care of any patient.
  - Not allow personal preference or bias to be a factor in the process of instruction and evaluation. If an instructor cannot perform an impartial evaluation on a particular student, she should request the program coordinator remove this student from her schedule.
  - Teach the student how, and when, to multitask. Multitasking is an essential competency for students. A student delegating skills (such as vital signs or breath sounds) while he takes medical histories is an example of failure to accomplish multitasking. Except in cases of necessity, delegations such as these will constitute unsatisfactory performance. A student asking his partner to set up an IV, or apply monitor leads, while he completes vital signs, breath sounds, and histories would be an example of effective multitasking. The instructor should use prompts to provide this instruction.
  - Do not substitute your own forms for those developed by the faculty of the program.
- Be specific when documenting unsatisfactory performance. "Prompt items" have been included in the various competencies of the critique forms. These items are designed to reduce the amount of writing an instructor has to do. Prompts can be documented by circling both the word "prompt" and the appropriate "prompt item" for that respective competency.
- Make the student verbalize. The instructor needs to know what the student is thinking at all times. This knowledge will allow the instructor to preempt potential student mistakes and oversights. The result will be improved care for the patient and less potential for liability for all EMS providers.

Receipt Page (for Instructors)

The guidelines included in this *Manual for Paramedic Students and Instructors* were developed, in part, to benefit instructors. This manual should be retained. It should serve as a reference guide for the paramedic instructor.

To: _____
             First   Middle initial   Last
                     (paramedic instructor)

Please print your name, sign your name, and write date of signature in the designated places. This page will be retained as verification that you have received a copy of the *Manual for Paramedic Students and Instructors.*

_____   Date: _____
(signature of paramedic instructor)

Witness: _____
                 (signature)
Title: _____   Date: _____
             (job title of witness)

Instructor: _____ **Station:** _____

Student: _____ **Time of arrival:** _____

1. Attire and Equipment   Satisfactory _____ Unsatisfactory _____
2. Equipment Checks   Satisfactory _____ Unsatisfactory _____ N/A _____
3. Documentation (logs)   Satisfactory _____ Unsatisfactory _____ N/A _____
4. Restocking   Satisfactory _____ Unsatisfactory _____ N/A _____
5. Cleaning/Maintenance   Satisfactory _____ Unsatisfactory _____ N/A _____
6. Completes self-study assignments Satisfactory _____ Unsatisfactory _____ N/A _____
7. Effectively uses down time   Satisfactory _____ Unsatisfactory _____ N/A _____
8. Relieved for end of shift   Satisfactory _____ Unsatisfactory _____
9. Affect/Professional Conduct   Satisfactory _____ Unsatisfactory _____

Instructor Comments:

_____

_____

_____

Student Comments:

_____

_____

_____

Signatures:

Instructor: _____ Date: _____

Student: _____ Date: _____

C Daily Log of Patient Contacts

These can be printed on a large envelope to secure critiques and other paperwork.

Date: _____ **Unit:** _____

Instructor: _____ **Student:** _____

Pt.	Incident #	Patient: Age, Sex, Complaint	TM/TL/TLE	Feedback
1				Y/N
2				Y/N
3				Y/N
4				Y/N
5				Y/N

Initials: Instructor: _____ Student: _____

Date: _____ **Unit:** _____

Instructor: _____ **Student:** _____

Pt.	Incident #	Patient: Age, Sex, Complaint	TM/TL/TLE	Feedback
1				Y/N
2				Y/N
3				Y/N
4				Y/N
5				Y/N

Initials: Instructor: _____ Student: _____

Date: _____   **Unit:** _____
Instructor: _____   **Student:** _____

Pt.	Incident #	Patient: Age, Sex, Complaint	TM/TL/TLE	Feedback
1				Y/N
2				Y/N
3				Y/N
4				Y/N
5				Y/N

Initials: Instructor: _____   Student: _____

Date: _____   **Unit:** _____
Instructor: _____   **Student:** _____

Pt.	Incident #	Patient: Age, Sex, Complaint	TM/TL/TLE	Feedback
1				Y/N
2				Y/N
3				Y/N
4				Y/N
5				Y/N

Initials: Instructor: _____   Student: _____

Date: _____   **Unit:** _____
Instructor: _____   **Student:** _____

Pt.	Incident #	Patient: Age, Sex, Complaint	TM/TL/TLE	Feedback
1				Y/N
2				Y/N
3				Y/N
4				Y/N
5				Y/N

Initials: Instructor: _____   Student: _____

D

FTO Quality Improvement

Two FTOs accompany the student. One FTO serves as the student's preceptor on the first patient contact, while the other FTO observes and critiques FTO/student interaction. On the second patient contact, the FTOs switch roles. Continue to alternate throughout the shift.

FTO Critique

Working FTO: _____ Date: _____

Observing FTO: _____ Location: _____

Student Name: _____ Phase: _____

Observing FTO should enter indicated data and circle appropriate information. Explain prompts by entering "comments."

Contact #1   Age/Sex of Patient: _____   Presentation: _____

Comments: _____

Prompts: Expectations   Positioning   Verbal Feedback   Prompting   Documentation   Affect

Student given score of: Satisfactory   Unsatisfactory

Agree/Disagree (with score)

Comments: _____

Contact #2   Age/Sex of Patient: _____   Presentation: _____

Comments: _____

Prompts: Expectations   Positioning   Verbal Feedback   Prompting   Documentation   Affect

Student given score of: Satisfactory   Unsatisfactory

Agree/Disagree (with score)

Comments: _____

Prepared for DTCC by EMS Education/Bayhealth Medical Center

Contact #3   Age/Sex of Patient: Presentation:

Comments: _____

Prompts: Expectations   Positioning   Verbal Feedback   Prompting   Documentation   Affect

Student given score of: Satisfactory   Unsatisfactory

Agree/Disagree (with score)

Comments: _____

_____

_____

_____

FTO: _____

_____

_____

_____

Observer: _____

_____

FTO signature: _____   Date: _____   Observer signature: _____

Notes:

Notes:

Notes:

Notes:

Notes:

www.ingramcontent.com/pod-product-compliance
Lightning Source LLC
Chambersburg PA
CBHW081532220326
41598CB00036B/6406